Maria do Livramento S. Bitencourt
Simone H. dos Santos Oliveira

Pressure Ulcers in the Intensive Care Unit

Maria do Livramento S. Bitencourt
Simone H. dos Santos Oliveira

Pressure Ulcers in the Intensive Care Unit

Incidence, prevalence and associated factors

ScienciaScripts

Imprint

Cover image: www.ingimage.com

This book is a translation from the original published under ISBN 978-613-9-64123-9.

Publisher:
Sciencia Scripts
is a trademark of
Dodo Books Indian Ocean Ltd. and OmniScriptum S.R.L publishing group

120 High Road, East Finchley, London, N2 9ED, United Kingdom
Str. Armeneasca 28/1, office 1, Chisinau MD-2012, Republic of Moldova, Europe
Printed at: see last page
ISBN: 978-620-7-72818-3

For from Him, and through Him, and for Him, are all
things; Glory therefore to Him eternally. Amen.

(ROMANS, 11:36)

THANKS

Above all and everyone I thank God, sovereign, kind, merciful, father, through Him and for Him are all things. There are no adjectives that can express my gratitude for You and Your love for my life; You are so great, but You care about me.

To my beloved and dear husband, who, despite complaining a lot, has an important role in my journey, often doing more than I thought possible;

To my beloved children, God's inheritance in my life, who even at the height of their adolescence knew how to understand my absence during this journey;

To my dear mother, an example of a warrior woman;

Especially to my sister Gorete, who followed this entire journey closely and always encouraged me and made me believe that I was capable;

To my Sister Raimunda (In memorian) who, even in her simplicity, encouraged me to go further and to all my brothers for their love and support;

I am especially grateful to my advisor, Professor **Simone Helena** , for the opportunity to participate in such a rich professional experience. Thank you for understanding and respecting my personal and professional limitations and my difficult moments. You are an example of a human being, woman, mother and professional. I am so grateful to God for putting you in my life and, especially, as my advisor. Once more, thank you;

To the professors and administrative technicians of the Postgraduate Program in Nursing (PPGENF), for the opportunity to complete this master's degree;

To Professor **Joab de Oliveira Lima** for his willingness, patience, dedication, simplicity and wisdom to welcome all those who seek his guidance;

To Professors **Gilson de Vasconcelos Torres, Maria Helena Lacher Caliri, Maria Júlia Guimarães Oliveira Soares and Marta Miriam Lopes Costa,** who promptly accepted the invitation to be part of the judging panel for this dissertation, contributing in an invaluable way to the final development of this study;

To the UFPB Nursing student, Rafaela do Ó Trindade, for her help in collecting data and for always being ready for any need.

To my friend **Edienne Rosângela** , inseparable companion. Without you everything would be much more difficult. You were very important on this journey. Your enthusiasm and optimism have contributed greatly to my learning;

To the Family that makes up the Military Police Hospital (HPM), especially the Administrative Director, in the person of **Maj. Bridges;** and to the General Nursing Supervisor, in the person of **Capt. Luciana** , for her understanding and support;

To all the staff at the Intensive Care Unit, I have immense affection for you, you are my second family;

To all the patients and family members without whom this project would not have been completed;

To the Nurse. **Jaciária** , faithful friend and companion, always willing to listen and encourage me;

To the skin commission in the people of Ten. **Sandra** , Nurses **Luana** and **Graça,** for always being ready to help me.

SUMMARY

CHAPTER 1

INTRODUCTION

The number of patients who acquire skin lesions after a long period of hospitalization has aroused the concern of health professionals, researchers and authorities on the subject, as it is a problem that, in most cases, can be avoidable and involves resulting in high costs for health institutions, in addition to causing physical and psychological suffering for the patient and their families (IRION, 2012).

Changes in the integrity of the skin that commonly result in pressure ulcers (UPP) have been reported as an object of nursing concern since its inception with Florence Nightingale (NOTAS..., 2010). However, the problem remains very present in hospital units and long-term care institutions, despite research results and technological advances developed to prevent and treat these injuries.

Pressure ulcers are defined as skin or soft tissue injuries basically caused by prolonged tissue ischemia. Any position maintained by a patient for a long period of time can cause tissue damage, especially in tissues that overlap a bony prominence, due to the presence of little subcutaneous tissue in these regions. Compression of these areas decreases local blood flow, facilitating the emergence of injury due to tissue ischemia and necrosis (WADA; NETO; FERREIRA, 2010; IRION, 2012).

According to Giovanini, Oliveira Júnior and Palermo (2007), the incidence of pressure ulcers reaches 10% in the United States and around 6% to 9% in European countries. In Brazil, studies have evaluated the incidence and prevalence of PU both in the hospital environment and in long-term care institutions and in homes, revealing that the numbers vary according to the setting and patient profile (GOMES et al., 2010; AGUIAR, 2011).

A study by Blanes et al., (2004), carried out at Hospital São Paulo (HSP), showed that 33.4% of PUs developed in the medical clinic, 28.2% in the emergency unit, 19.2% in the surgical clinic and the same percentage for the intensive care unit.

In a university hospital in Natal-RN, Paiva (2008) found that among the patients who developed PU, 16.7% were admitted to the wards, without specifying whether clinical or surgical; same percentage for ICU; 6.7% for the ICU/Infirmary sector and 3.3% for neurology, showing an overall incidence in the hospital of 43.3%, with 83.3% in the ICU, 38.5% in the wards, 33.3 % in the ICU/ENF and 20% in neurology.

In the intensive care environment, the occurrence of UPP can present with even higher numbers, due to the severity of the patients, frequent therapeutic procedures, immobility in bed, connection of specific devices, loss of muscle mass and long periods of hospitalization (FERNANDES; TORRES; VIEIRA, 2008).

In a prospective study, carried out by Cremasco et al. (2009), in three ICUs of a university hospital in the city of São Paulo - SP, an incidence of 31% for pressure ulcers was identified. Fernandes and Torres (2006) identified a 50% incidence in ICUs in private hospitals in Rio Grande do Norte. And Gomes et al., (2010)

35.2% in a study carried out in fifteen ICUs in public and private hospitals in Minas Gerais - MG.

In João Pessoa-PB, researchers from the Wound Treatment Study and Research Group (GEPEFE), when carrying out a study with patients with UPP in the medical, surgical and intensive care unit sectors of a university hospital, found that, of the fourteen patients who developed the injury, seven were admitted to the ICU (ARAÚJO et al., 2010).

Lindohlm (2007) states that pressure ulcers are between the third and fourth most expensive health problems in the world, being seen as an economic problem for health services. However, a significant reduction and improvement in the quality of life of sufferers can be achieved by deepening knowledge, creating guidelines and using specific methods and processes for prevention. The author also mentions that a community in Sweden managed to reduce ulcers by half in just one year, thus turning every dollar spent on preventing this problem into ten dollars in gains in terms of public health.

Corroborating, Rodrigues, Souza and Silva (2008) mention that most PUs can be preventable and that, in many countries, research shows that the costs of prevention are much lower than those spent on treatment. However, this is a major challenge, as, in practice, many barriers have been encountered that make it difficult to resolve this problem, such as: the lack of a common language in terms of risk factors, different understanding of professionals in relation to UPP , the lack of material resources that can improve preventive practice, in addition to the work overload that has been subjected to professionals, especially nursing professionals, which ends up making it difficult to carry out simple and economical measures such as repositioning the patient in bed in scheduled times (LOURO; FERREIRA; PÓVOA, 2007; IRION, 2012).

Given the risk that hospitalized patients, especially in ICUs, present for the development of UPP, researchers and health professionals have been seeking to develop strategies that prevent this condition and give professionals responsibility for improving the quality of care (WOCN, 2010).

Irion (2012) endorses that, in addition to the ethical issues involving the prevention of ulcers, in the USA, for example, the Center For Medicare and Medicaid Services (CMS) will no longer provide extra payments for the treatment of UPPs that were not yet installed in the at the time of hospital admission, that is, the institution will have to bear all the expenses caused by the treatment of the injuries.

In this scope, preventing UPP constitutes a challenge for health professionals and especially for the nursing team, as they maintain greater contact with the patient and are primarily responsible for assessing the risks to which they are exposed. and for planning and implementing preventive measures, as well as, together with the multidisciplinary team, being involved in making decisions about the most appropriate therapeutic measures for the treatment of PU at different stages, considering the patient's clinical conditions.

Santos et al., (2007) endorse that nursing has assumed an extremely important role in the process of caring for wounds, acting in prevention, treatment, clinical research and the development of new alternatives to intervene with patients at risk or with UPP installed.

This context requires nursing's continuous search for knowledge, striving to remain up to date on this problem, as well as to diagnose risks and identify alternatives that can be inserted in different realities, in order to prevent and treat these injuries, using existing advances, with a view to reducing the incidence of pressure ulcers.

With this aim, we seek to be included in the Study and Research Group on Wound Treatment - GEPEFE/PPGENF/UFPB, whose participation has allowed us to deepen our knowledge about the complex problem that involves the prevention and care of patients with wounds, in particularly those with chronic wounds such as pressure ulcers and has also reaffirmed the need to increasingly base nursing actions on diagnoses of health problems in different contexts, which can be favored by the development of scientific investigations.

I have been a nurse for fifteen years, working in a public hospital institution as a support worker in the medical and surgical clinical sectors and for ten years in the intensive care unit and, living with the occurrence of UPPs on a daily basis, I felt the need to carry out a study to evaluate the extent of the development of UPP in our practice and also to support the care provided to our patients.

Therefore, together with a group of nurses from the institution, a preliminary study was carried out through a retrospective search in the medical records of patients admitted to the hospital, over a period of one year. In this case, the findings proved to be peculiar to each sector investigated. In the Intensive Care Unit - ICU, for example, the prevalence of PU was 17.1%, which drew attention to the pressing need to propose measures to reduce the occurrence of this condition, since these numbers may still be greater when considering the possibility of underreporting of records. (OLIVEIRA et al., 2011).

This preliminary study, although it revealed significant information about the problem in the institution and particularly in the ICU, due to being a retrospective research in which records in the medical records were considered, did not reveal relevant information obtained, for example, during the physical examination, the meticulous assessment of the skin, existing lesions and other risk factors, which result from the daily monitoring of patients, which serve as a basis for a review of the preventive and treatment procedures adopted in the institution to date.

In view of the above and aware of the responsibility as local ICU manager, supported by the guidelines that state that the first step is to know the reality of a problem and then act and, also, given the complexity of the UPP problem for the patient, family members, professionals health and institution, we propose to carry out this investigation, seeking an answer to the following question: what is the incidence, prevalence and factors associated with pressure ulcers in intensive care units?

Thus, we hope to outline an overview of the UPP in our reality, providing health professionals with subsidies to support the request for technological resources to intervene in this problem with better resolution, increasing prevention and consequently reducing the institution's costs arising from treatment and the possible need longer hospital stay.

We also hope to draw the attention of professionals and institution managers to the problem, making them aware of the need for professional training, implementation of prophylactic measures for UPP and, mainly, the provision of integrated care to patients and their families.

CHAPTER 2

GOALS

2.1 Main goal:

To analyze the incidence, prevalence and factors associated with pressure ulcers in an intensive care unit.

2.2 Specific objectives:

> Identify the incidence and prevalence of pressure ulcers in patients admitted to the intensive care unit of a public hospital in João Pessoa - PB;

> Check the risk for developing UPP in patients, using the Braden Scale;

> To verify the association of sociodemographic and clinical data and risk factors with the presence of pressure ulcers among intensive care unit patients.

> Analyze the association of Braden subscale risk scores with the occurrence of pressure ulcers;

CHAPTER 3

LITERATURE REVIEW

3.1 PRESSURE ULCER (UPP) AND VULNERABILITIES OF PATIENTS ADMITTED TO THE INTENSIVE CARE UNIT (ICU)

Pressure ulcers are the name given to wounds caused by tissue damage within accommodation surfaces and bony prominences (IRION, 2012). It occurs when interstitial pressure exceeds intracapillary pressure, causing a reduction in blood flow and, consequently, oxygen and nutrients to cells, causing cell death (WADA; NETO; FERREIRA, 2010).

Going through the literature on the subject, it is possible to find different definitions by different authors about pressure ulcers, but they all refer to the definition of the National Pressure Ulcer Advisory Panel (NPUAP), considered one of the most accepted, which defines it as a localized area of cell death, which develops when the skin and/or soft tissue is compressed under a bony prominence as a result of pressure or a combination of pressure with friction and shear (NPUAP, 2009).

The occurrence of UPP related to the vulnerability of patients hospitalized in an intensive care environment understands the severity of the clinical condition which, in general, leads to frequent malnutrition, reduced mobility and the need for many connected devices, which in turn reduce the patient's ability to tolerate skin to pressure and shear, which makes these patients more prone to the risk of acquiring PU than those in other wards of the same institution (IRION, 2012).

The intensive care unit is a hospital area intended for patients in critical condition, who require highly complex care and frequent and rigorous controls (GOMES, 2011). It is a specialized environment, both in human potential and in equipment, whose primary function is to restore health and life through the combination of medical and nursing care in caring for seriously ill patients (SILVA et al., 2009).

A seriously ill patient is one who presents instability in one or more vital organs, who threatens to present some hemodynamic alteration or has serious clinical conditions associated with the need for invasive or non-invasive therapies of great complexity (CARDOSO; CALIRI; HASS, 2004). For Fernandes and Torres (2008), the ICU is the ideal place for the treatment of critically ill patients, although it is also one of the most hostile environments in the hospital which, associated with other factors, such as unfavorable sleep conditions, submission to procedures frequent therapies, absence from family, long stay in bed, fear of worsening of the condition and death, contribute to the emergence of complications such as muscular atrophy and PU.

In this scope, Mattia et al., (2010) mention that unfavorable clinical conditions expose patients to complications, including pressure ulcers, with repercussions on morbidity and mortality. Moro et al., (2007) add that these injuries represent one of the main complications that affect critically ill hospitalized patients.

Fernandes and Caliri (2000) mention that patients under intensive care are more susceptible to the development of PU due to sedation, altered level of consciousness, use of mechanical ventilation and vasoactive drugs, prolonged immobility and hemodynamic instability.

Patients admitted to an intensive care unit generally present a severe clinical condition, which can trigger organ failure, which in turn causes a drop in blood pressure and cardiac output and consequently a decrease in skin perfusion. Corroborating this, unsatisfactory positioning in bed and edema cause a reduction in the ability to transport nutrients to the skin and, together, all these factors increase the likelihood of skin lesions occurring (IRION, 2012).

In this context, UPP are configured as an alteration of the integrity of the skin and a significant complication, which may arise in patients hospitalized in critical environments, such as the ICU, mainly due to their conditions of restriction to the bed, presentation of hemodynamic instability, limitation of movements due to pathologies, thus characterizing a high risk for the formation of these injuries (MAIA; MONTEIRO, 2011).

Beneficial for the seriously ill client, but harmful for presenting several adverse situations, the intensive care environment increases the incidence and prevalence of PU to higher numbers than in other hospital wards (IRION, 2012).

3.1.1 Risk factors for pressure ulcers

All circumstances that expose the patient to long intervals of tissue ischemia caused by pressure and that reduce the tissue's ability to repair must be considered and evaluated as risk factors for the development of pressure ulcers (WADA; NETO; FERREIRA, 2010) .

The possible risks for the occurrence of PU are generally associated with immobility, lack of cognition/motivation to move in bed and other situations that, alone or in combination, favor the appearance of these injuries (IRION, 2012).

Braden and Bergstrom (1987) point out the intensity and duration of pressure and the tissue tolerance to withstand this pressure as being the most critical factors for the development of UPP. They also describe the presence of internal/intrinsic/primary and external/extrinsic/secondary factors as supporting factors in this process.

Intrinsic factors are those inherent to the individual that involve systemic and local conditions including loss of sensitivity and decreased muscle strength or mobility, fecal and urinary incontinence, hematopoietic changes, protein malnutrition, smoking, comorbidities, inadequate tissue perfusion and advanced age. The extrinsic ones consist of pressure, friction and shear, associated with humidity (SOUZA; SANTOS, 2007; MATTIA et al., 2010).

When pressure is applied continuously to a certain body area, it obstructs blood vessels and progresses to edema and occlusion of capillaries and lymphatics. When patients have preserved sensitivity and movement, they move, relieving the pressure, before it causes an injury, but, without repositioning, it can trigger thrombosis of capillaries and occlusion of the venous network, causing a vicious circle of edema and occlusion (IRION, 2012).

Friction is generated when two surfaces are rubbed together. Its effects can be worsened in the presence of humidity and occurs when the patient is dragged instead of lifted from the bed, removing the outer layers of epithelial cells (SILVA et al., 2011).

Shear generally occurs in individuals who are sitting or lying down with a decubitus position greater than 30 degrees for a long period of time. It reaches tissues deeper than friction and distorts blood vessels leading to ischemia in the injured tissue, which is why it is a greater risk factor (IRION, 2012).

3.1.1 Assessment and stratification of risk for pressure ulcers

Studies show that the costs of treating PU are very high, leaving prevention as a more economical alternative, which begins with the need to assess the risk that the patient presents for developing PU, know the risk factors to which they are exposed and the preventive measures available in the unit to then implement a care plan aimed at preventing this condition.

NPUAP (2009) recommends that each institution establish a risk assessment policy that includes a structured approach in the following items: identification of the most critical sectors for risk, determination of the assessment and reassessment time for each client, recording of the assessment and that all information is accessible to all healthcare professionals.

The structured approach to risk assessment must include the meticulous examination of skin conditions, the professional's clinical judgment, the insertion of a predictive scale and recording of all assessments, and must be carried out as soon as the patient is admitted, repeated regularly and with the frequency required by the individual's health condition (NPUAP, 2009). For Fernandes and Caliri (2008), assessing the risk for UPP should be the first approach adopted for prevention.

Still seeking to identify patients at risk for developing UPP, one must consider those with dry skin, non-blanchable erythema and other changes, as well as those restricted to bed and/or confined to wheelchairs. (NPUAP, 2009).

According to Wocn (2010), risk assessment must be carried out when the patient is admitted to the service and repeated at regular periods or when there is a significant change in the patient's general condition. For Moro et al., (2007) the assessment should be carried out within the first six hours of the patient's admission to the unit, with reassessment recommended only after the next forty-eight hours. For Gomes et al., (2009), the first assessment must take place between twelve and twenty-four hours after admission and the reassessment every twelve hours, emphasizing that it must occur holistically.

We agree that the assessment of the risk for the development of UPP must occur at the time of admission, immediately after stabilization of the clinical condition, planning the relevant interventions as soon as possible, in order to prevent the appearance of the lesions.

Even though there are disagreements between the authors regarding the best time to carry out the risk assessment for PU, everyone agrees that it should be carried out to assist in the implementation of appropriate prophylactic measures. Corroborating, Silva et al., (2011) mention that in studies in which risk assessment was formally inserted and the risk levels obtained were referred to prevention protocols, the incidence of PU reduced by 60%, accompanied by a reduction severity and costs of care.

In addition to risk assessment and considering the ethical and legal implications involving the problem of UPP, it is extremely important to record the presence of these injuries, their stages and characteristics during the patient's admission (BRANDÃO; SANTOS; SANTOS, 2011).

3.1.2 Instruments for risk stratification

When browsing books and research articles, it is possible to find several instruments that can be used to help professionals measure the risk presented by the patient for developing PU. However, it is known that the instrument to be used in a given group of patients must be compatible with their reality and have its sensitivity and specificity extensively tested, proving its effectiveness and ease of application by the professionals who will use it (ROCHA ; BARROS, 2007).

Brandão, Santos and Santos (2011) add that the instrument to be used to measure the risk for the development of UPP must be chosen by the nurse responsible for the service, who must look for the one that is most appropriate to the reality of the sector and the profile of the patients. patients served.

For Falci and Cruz (2008), the use of predictive risk scales adds the accuracy and effectiveness of the nurse's intervention and should be the first requirement to be included in clinical practice manuals or prevention protocols.

The use of scales to predict the risk for PU, associated with the patient's clinical and social history, can benefit the nurse and other members of the multidisciplinary team in planning care actions (AGUIAR, 2011).

In this sense, the Braden, Norton, Gosnell and Wartelow scales are the best known and applied in research, with the Braden scale being the most used, as it has the best functional definition and proved to have greater sensitivity and specificity in relation to the others, in addition to being indicated for use in older adults, clinically and cognitively involved, which is similar to the profile of patients admitted to the ICU (SERPA, 2006; AYELLO, 2007; GOMES et al., 2010).

In this context, Gomes et al. (2009), when carrying out a bibliographical research on publications from 1996 to 2007, they showed that the Braden Scale is the instrument of choice for evaluating patients regarding the risk of developing PU because it is easy to apply, widely researched and known. by health professionals.

In a case study carried out in Paraná by Ito et al., (2004), using the Braden Scale to measure the risk of PU when using a Monitoring Protocol for critically ill patients, they obtained only one episode of injury onset, demonstrating that the protocol was effective in reducing the incidence of PU in patients admitted to a critical care unit.

In Texas (USA), in a cohort study carried out by Fife et al., (2001), the risk factors for the development of UPP were addressed using the Braden scale as a predictor of this risk in seriously ill patients, proving that This instrument is a preliminary predictor of the risk of developing PU in this population, especially in those with low weight.

For Fernandes and Torres (2008), the Braden Scale appears as an effective instrument to assist nurses in prophylactic interventions, according to the individual risk of each client.

The Braden Scale was created by Bergston, Braden, Laguzza and Holman in 1987 and validated in Brazil by Paranhos and Santos (1999), adapting and testing its predictive validity in 34 patients in an intensive care unit. The scale was created to guide nursing procedures aimed at preventing PU and consequently reducing its incidence. Its construction was based on the pathophysiology of the injury, considering items determining its development, such as: intensity and duration of pressure on the tissues and tolerance of the skin and adjacent structures to support it. In Brazil, it is the most used by nurses to measure the risk of PU (SILVA et al., 2011).

In total, the scale contains six parameters or subscales. Three are related to clinical determinants of pressure exposure, such as activity, mobility and sensory perception, understood as: ability to change, maintain or sustain certain body positions; ability to remove any pressure on areas of the skin/body, promoting circulation; and level of consciousness that reflects the individual's ability to perceive painful stimuli or discomfort and react by making changes in position or requesting help to carry them out (ANSELMI; PREDUZZI; JÚNIOR, 2009). The other three parameters evaluate the tissue's tolerance to pressure - humidity, nutrition, friction and shear, understood as: degree of humidity to which the skin is exposed; usual feeding pattern and the way the patient is moved or repositioned in bed (GOMES; MAGALHÃES, 2008).

3.1.3 Assessment of pressure ulcers

The evaluation of pressure ulcers encompasses clinical judgment, patient history and direct observation by the professional who, together with other instruments and techniques, can gather information about the anatomical location; evolution time; sizing in terms of diameter and depth; characteristics of the wound bed, such as the presence of granulation or necrotic tissue, fistulas, tunnels and inflammatory signs; appearance of the exudate; odor; appearance of neighboring skin and classification regarding the level of tissue involvement (stage, degree, category) (IRION, 2012).

The initial assessment must occur in an adequate, holistic way, to provide support for designing the treatment and evaluating the results, in addition to promoting communication between the professionals involved (AHCPR, 1992).

According to Costa (2010), a reduction in the incidence of PU can be achieved if the patient is assessed for risk upon admission and if there is continuity in subsequent assessments.

For adequate action or intervention, reassessment must occur at least once a week. Everything must be recorded. Color photographic records must be taken to help monitor the lesion's response to treatment, as long as the patient authorizes it (WOCN, 2010).

Regarding the anatomical location of UPP, research reports that the most affected areas are the sacral region, trochanter and calcaneus, as these are areas of bony prominences that are most exposed to the effects of pressure, friction and shear, preponderant factors in the formation of injuries (MATOS; DUARTE; MINETO, 2010;

To measure the size of the wound, Silva et al., (2011) recommend that measurements be taken by the same evaluator, using the same techniques and instruments, always keeping the patient in the same position, to avoid errors in collecting information. In addition, Irion (2012) states that the size of the wound generally changes little while it remains infected.

From the perspective of various instruments, such as rulers, graph paper, sterile swab or probe and applicator with a cotton tip (placed vertically at the deepest point of the lesion) and techniques that can be used to measure the wound, the use of **from the base of the clock where the "cephalic direction on the trunk and the proximal direction on a limb** as 12:00 h and the **caudal direction on the trunk or distal direction on a limb as 6:00 h"** (IRION, 2012 p. 117). Thus, the length refers to the space between 12 and 06 o'clock and the width from 09 to 03 o'clock. Another method described in the literature consists of measuring the greatest length and width without being related to the shape of the wound. Whichever technique is used, the length is multiplied by the width to measure the diameter of the ulcer and the result is subject to greater or lesser errors depending on the shape of the wound (IRION, 2012).

According to the damage observed and considering the affected structures, there are several methods to classify pressure ulcers, but the most used is the one proposed by the American National Pressure Ulcer Advisory Panel (NPUAP) and European Pressure Ulcer Advisory Panel (EPUAP) which, in their latest update, they present a suggestion to replace the terms used until then (stage, degree) which, according to experts, such words suggest a hierarchy, and may indicate a progression or cure from I to IV or from IV to I, when neither is always the case. Thus, the two organizations reached a consensus that **they should use a neutral term to classify the UPPs and indicated the word "category".** However, they emphasize that it is not wrong to use the previous terms, and it is up to professionals to choose the one that comes closest to their reality. In this update, they also added two more categories to their classification, establishing them as follows: category I, **II, III, IV, suspected deep tissue injury and "non-stageable" ulcer (NPUAP, 2009).**

Category I : intact skin, showing hyperemia in a specific area that does not whiten after removing the pressure, generally over a bony prominence. In people with dark skin it can be difficult to detect due to the difficulty in noticing the whitening. The affected area is generally painful, hardened or softened, hotter or colder when compared to neighboring tissues (NPUAP, 2009).

Category II: injury involving partial loss of the epidermis, dermis or both. It presents as a superficial ulcer with a pinkish bed, without slough. Its appearance is that of a blister containing serous exudate, which may be intact or ruptured. When there is slough or purpleness of the tissue, it will suggest deep tissue injury (NPUAP, 2009).

Category III: characterized by full-thickness skin loss, involving damage or necrosis of the subcutaneous tissue. It may be deep depending on its anatomical location, but without affecting muscles, tendons or bones. There may be the presence of slough, but without hindering the identification of the depth of tissue loss. It is possible to contain detachments and tunnels (NPUAP, 2009).

Category IV : full thickness skin loss with extensive destruction, damaging muscles, bones, or other support structures such as tendons or joints. There may be slough or eschar in some parts of the wound bed. Often includes undermining and tunneling. Its depth also varies depending on the affected region of the body. The display of bone or tendon is apparent or palpable (NPUAP, 2009).

For injuries that do not fit into these categories, we suspect deep tissue injury and pressure ulcers that cannot be classified (not measurable). The first **characteristic** is characterized by the identification of a localized area of intact skin, purple or brown in color, or a bloody blister, caused by damage to the soft tissue, resulting from pressure and/or shear. The site is usually preceded by a painful, hardened or softened, spongy tissue that has a different temperature compared to the adjacent tissue. In dark-skinned individuals, this type of lesion becomes difficult to identify. Its evolution may include a fine blister over the dark wound bed and become covered by a thin eschar. It runs the risk of progressing quickly with exposure of additional tissue layers even with adequate treatment (NPUAP, 2009).

Ulcers that cannot be classified are characterized by total loss of tissue, with the base covered by a yellow, brown, gray, greenish or brown crust, or by eschar that appears brown, brown or black. Its classification will only occur after debridement has been carried out, which exposes the base of the lesion, making it possible to identify the depth of tissue damage. When it appears as a stable eschar (dry, adherent, intact, without erythema or fluctuation) on the heels, it functions as **a "biological covering of the body" and should not be removed (NPUAP, 2009). After classifying the ulcer category,** it is maintained until it heals, that is, it does not reduce even with regression in the depth of the lesion. Scar by secondary intention as it is covered by granulation tissue and its assessment must be made by measuring its size (GOMES; MAGALHÃES, 2008).

3.2 PREVENTIVE STRATEGIES FOR PRESSURE ULCERS

Preventive measures are strategies adopted in the present aiming at future results, guiding diagnoses and actions to provide assistance and improve quality of life (RODRIGUES; SOUZA; SILVA, 2008). Analyzing the pathophysiology of PU, the authors state that prevention is the best way to provide care (FALCI; CRUZ, 2008; FERNANDES; CALIRI; HAAS, 2008).

The international community composed of the American National Pressure Ulcer Advisory Panel and the European Pressure Ulcer Advisory Panel, after extensive discussion, organized in 2009 an update of guidelines based on clinical evidence and expert consensus for managing the prevention and treatment of PU, to be applied by all health professionals to patients and/or people vulnerable to the risk of developing pressure ulcers, whether in a hospital, long-term care institution or any other care environment, regardless of their clinical diagnosis (NPUAP; EPUAP, 2009).

Considering that pressure ulcers are unpleasant complications that affect patients and families and that, according to Rocha, Miranda and Andrade (2006), the adoption of preventive measures, in addition to establishing an effective approach, significantly reduces the risk of their development, recommends - follow the NPUAP and EPUAP guidelines, which, based on clinical evidence and expert consensus, guide the management of prevention and treatment of PU, highlighting the main strategies:

Skin assessment - NPUAP (2009) recommends that every institution should include in its risk assessment a structured approach to examining skin that includes: professional training to identify non-bleaching, local heat, hardening or softening; guide the patient to mention areas of discomfort or pain that may be associated with the effects of pressure suffered by the tissues; and also specific care for the skin, such as not placing it on an area that is already hyperemic, not massaging or rubbing areas that are at risk of UPP, hydrating and protecting it from excessive humidity. Every skin assessment must be continuous and documented to monitor the patient's progress and for communication between professionals.

Skin surveillance should be daily, mainly focused on bony prominences and other body regions exposed to pressure from medical devices such as probes, masks and catheters (CUERVO, 2008).

Nutrition to prevent pressure ulcers - since malnutrition is a risk factor for PU, all individuals at risk must have their nutritional status assessed so that interventions can be anticipated in advance of the development of the condition. The recommendation is to use a valid, reliable and practical instrument for nutritional screening that is easy to use by the health professional (NPUAP, 2009).

Those identified at nutritional risk and for UPP should be referred to a nutritionist and, if necessary, to a multidisciplinary nutritional team; receive nutritional support through protein-rich supplements, administered at regular meal intervals so as not to reduce the food intake already established; consume at least 30 to 35 calories per kilogram of body weight per day, and 1.25 to 1.50 grams of protein per kilogram per day (NPUAP, 2009).

Recommendations for repositioning in bed - pressure ulcer prevention measures are relatively simple and inexpensive. The most important basic measure is the periodic change of the patient's positioning. Relieving pressure on a bony prominence for 5 minutes every 2 hours allows adequate tissue recovery from ischemic aggression and often prevents the formation of the lesion. It is important when changing the patient's position to avoid movements that cause friction or shearing of the skin (WADA; NETO; FERREIRA, 2010).

With level of evidence (A), bed repositioning should be considered for all patients at risk of PU, in order to reduce the duration and magnitude of pressure on susceptible areas of the body (NPUAP, 2009).

It is extremely important to reduce the time and amount of pressure exerted on a specific, most vulnerable area, since tissue damage can occur using either high pressure for a short period of time or low pressure for a long period of time (NPUAP, 2009) . Thus, the panel of American experts recommends that before determining intervals for changing position, one should evaluate the patient's clinical conditions and treatment objectives, support surface being used, tissue tolerance, ability to move in bed, as well as the characteristics of the skin and the individual's general comfort.

To perform the repositioning technique, follow the following items: place the patient in a position that relieves or redistributes pressure; never expose the skin to pressure and shear forces, therefore, do not drag, suspend the individual while repositioning him; avoid positioning over bony prominences, non-blanchable areas and over medical devices (probes, drains); use 30 degrees for the semi-fowler, pronation and right and left lateralization positions (NPUAP, 2009).

Finally, select a posture that is comfortable and acceptable to the patient, minimizing the pressure and shear exerted on the skin and soft tissues and record the plan established for repositioning in bed, especially the frequency, the position adopted, impediments, if any, and evaluate the results of this plan (NPUAP, 2009).

Provide training on the equipment available in the unit and the use of repositioning techniques to prevent PU, for professionals involved in care and, if possible, for the patient and caregiver (NPUAP, 2009).

Support surface - from this perspective, the industry has produced many equipment and materials that can be considered reducers or relief devices that redistribute the pressure suffered by tissues to other areas with greater tolerance to support it, providing pressure reduction in areas of greater risk of being injured (ASSOCIAÇÃO AMIGOS DA GRANDE IDADE, 2012). They must be used according to the individual needs of each patient and provide an interface pressure of 26 to 32 mmHg (IRION, 2012).

Health professionals need to know the support surfaces available in their service, be able to use and carry out maintenance, in order to achieve success in their application and durability of the equipment (ASSOCIAÇÃO AMIGOS DA GRANDE IDADE, 2012).

The NPUAP (2009) mentions that to choose an adequate support surface, one must consider the patient's degree of mobility in bed, their comfort, the location and conditions for providing care, also checking whether the support surface is compatible with the treatment environment.

It also recommends checking the useful life of support surfaces, giving preference to highly specific foams, using protective devices on the heels that keep them elevated from the bed, but without putting pressure on the Achilles tendon, not using mattresses or alternating pressure overlaps with small cells and giving special attention to spinal cord injured patients (NPUAP, 2009). Below is a description of some products found on the market to prevent PU in both hospital and home environments:

Mattress replacements - designed to fit the standardized bed frame, replacing the traditional mattress. They can be air, foam, gel or water. When made of foam (which are the most common) they must have a density greater than 28.8 kg/m ^{3} , delaying excessive deformation and premature fatigue of the foam. Currently, the market offers mattresses with alternating compression, with low air loss, and associated characteristics (IRION, 2012). The AHCPR (1992) recommendation is to use dynamic accommodation surfaces for those patients who are unable to adopt a change in body position, and static accommodation surfaces when the patient adopts different positions.

Pillows/Cushions/Rollers - the use of these devices relieves pressure on bony protrusions such as heels, malleoli and knees and also helps to reposition the patient in bed (CÂNDIDO, 2010).

In this preventive context of UPP, some coverings are described in the literature as supporting this process, highlighting: **hydrocolloid** - its outer layer is composed of film or polyurethane foam, impermeable to water and microorganisms; the internal part is based on gelatin, pectin and carboxymethylcellulose. Indicated for the prevention of areas considered to be at higher risk and also for the treatment of UPP that present certain clinical characteristics (SILVA et al., 2011).

Transparent/semi-permeable membrane or film - composed of polyurethane, transparent, impermeable to fluids and microorganisms and adhesive to dry skin. Indicated for the prevention of category I UPP, to fix and protect vascular catheters from contamination, protection of the skin surrounding wounds with exudate and as covers for intact incisions (SILVA et al., 2011). A clinical research carried out by Souza (2010) analyzed the effectiveness of transparent polyurethane film for preventing UPP in heels and found a significantly lower incidence in the group that underwent the intervention.

The devices are used to aid prevention and as a fundamental complement to treatment, but do not replace the need for regular and patient-appropriate repositioning (ROCHA; MIRANDA; ANDRADE, 2006). Some simple and economically viable measures can be used in both hospital and home environments, such as, for example, keeping the skin clean, free from moisture and hydrated with natural oils, using absorbent diapers and controlling excess pressure on bony prominences by protecting them. with pressure relievers/reducers that redistribute body weight and reduce pressure (LISE; SILVA, 2007).

CHAPTER 4

METHOD

4.1 Kind of study

This is a descriptive study, with a quantitative approach. According to Moreira and Caleffe (2006), descriptive research has its value based on the premise that problems can be solved and practices improved through objective and detailed observation of analysis and description.

4.2 Search location

The research was carried out in an ICU of a medium-sized public hospital in João Pessoa-PB, which is intended to provide general care to the population of João Pessoa and other municipalities in the state of Paraíba. The ICU has seven beds and receives clinical and surgical patients from the hospital itself or referred by the state regulatory system.

In relation to the human resources of the unit, it has ten doctors on duty and a coordinator, six nurses on duty and a coordinator, thirty nursing technicians, a physiotherapist and a speech therapist on duty. Nutritionists, psychologists and social workers carry out daily visits to the unit.

Nursing care is based on the SAE (Nursing Care Systematization) based on the theory of Basic Human Needs by Wanda de Aguiar Horta. To collect and record the information, a form prepared in the form of a checklist is used, which is completed by the nurse, responsible for carrying out all phases of the care process, and the nursing technicians are responsible for carrying out the prescribed care and recording it on the form. The checklist contains a summarized copy of the Braden Scale, for the nurse to assess the risk for the development of PU and a table for recording the PU, describing their location and stage of evolution, when the injury is present.

It is worth highlighting the presence of the Skin Committee at the institution, which operates in all units. It is made up of three nurses and three nursing technicians. In the ICU, there is a nurse and a nursing technician who, from Monday to Friday, carry out prevention and treatment interventions that require specific materials, such as the application of polyurethane films, hydrocolloid plates and foams in areas of prominence, and They perform UPP dressings or other more complex procedures (infected or dehisced dressings) in the morning, generally during bed baths, a suitable time for identifying injured or at-risk areas. The actions adopted and the results are shared with other members of the healthcare team.

Considering the severity of patients hospitalized in an intensive care environment and the risk factors to which they are exposed and, based on the understanding that UPP are unpleasant complications that can favor other illnesses and that prevention is the most economical resource, it is considered extremely It is important to invest in the prevention of these skin lesions. Therefore, management has focused on raising awareness among professionals about the issue, with two workshops on the issue being held in the hospital institution's auditorium over the last six months.

Concerning the routines adopted in the unit to prevent UPP, these generally involve simple procedures that are under the responsibility of the nursing team and include measures such as repositioning the bed at scheduled times and according to the patient's clinical conditions, suspending the patient supported by a cross member to avoid dragging it; hydrating the skin with common moisturizers and oils (Essential Fatty Acids); skin protection with the use of absorbent diapers and barrier cream; maintaining clean, dry skin and clean, stretched sheets. We currently have a variety of products suitable for use on injuries that develop in the ICU or that, during admission, are already present. However, the most recent and perhaps important strategy for preventing UPP was the acquisition of pneumatic mattresses (dynamic air) for all beds, which were put into use in July 2012.

4.3 Population and sample

The study population consisted of all patients admitted to the ICU of that institution, from July to October 2012. To calculate the sample size, the three months prior to data collection were taken as a basis. Thus, in the months of April, May

and June 2012, 89 patients were admitted to the hospital's ICU. The preliminary retrospective study on the prevalence of UPP in that unit identified a prevalence of 17.1% (OLIVEIRA et al., 2011).

Therefore, a universe of 89 patients was considered with a proportion of 17.1% of an individual in this universe developing UPP, a maximum sampling error of 8% and a significance level for statistical tests of 5%. Thus, based on this information, the sample size calculation ***(ri)*** can be obtained in the following way (CAMPBELL; STANLEY, 1979):

$$n \geq \frac{Np(1-p)}{(N-1)\left(\frac{Erro}{z_{\alpha/2}}\right)^2 + p(1-p)}$$

On what:

ne is the minimum sample size that should be selected;

N: is the population size;

p: is the proportion, within the population, of a key study variable. In the case of this study, ***p*** is the proportion of patients occurring in May/2012;

Error is the maximum allowable error that the researcher is willing to assume for the results that will be extracted from the sample.

$z_{\alpha/2}$: is the $\alpha/2$ level percentile of a Normal Distribution.

Thus, the calculation for the minimum sample size resulted in:

$$n \geq \frac{89 \times 0{,}171 \times 0{,}829}{(88)\left(\frac{0{,}07}{1{,}96}\right)^2 + 0{,}171 \times 0{,}829} \geq 44$$

Having defined the sample size, the following inclusion criteria were chosen: being aged 18 years or over, remaining hospitalized in the unit for a minimum period of twenty-four hours, being subjected to at least two assessments and consenting to participate in the research or have it authorized by their legal guardian, by signing the Free and Informed Consent Form - ICF (Appendix II). Thus, during the data collection period, 57 patients were admitted to the ICU, resulting in a sample of 45 participants that met the inclusion criteria, as described in Figure 1:

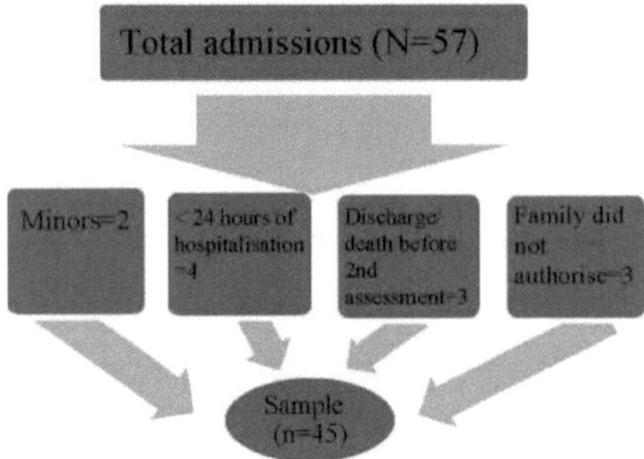

Figure 1- Sample selection flowchart.

Source: Direct research. João Pessoa — PB, 2013.

4.4 Data collection instruments and procedures

To achieve the objectives outlined, data collection was carried out using instruments and procedures relevant to each moment of the research. In order to facilitate understanding, the implementation phases and the respective instruments and procedures adopted in each of them are presented below.

First phase: initial assessment

To collect data in this phase of the research, two instruments were used, a form and a predictive scale of risk for PU. The form was structured into three parts: the first intended for recording the patient's sociodemographic data; the second, to clinical data relevant to the development of pressure ulcers and the third, covering the physical examination and assessment of skin conditions (Appendix III).

To estimate the risk of developing PU, we chose the Braden Scale, an instrument constructed by Bergstom et al., (1987) and validated in Brazil by Paranhos and Santos (1999) (Appendix III). Although it was not created specifically for use in seriously ill patients, it has been widely used by nurses and researchers, as it presents greater specificity and sensitivity in this population. (PARANHOS; SANTOS, 1999). According to Fernandes and Caliri (2008), it is an instrument that can be used by nurses to estimate the risk to which each patient is exposed, helping to implement the preventive measures indicated for each case.

The scale provides six parameters or subscales to assess the risk of PU, such as: 1- sensory perception; 2- humidity; 3- activity; 4- mobility; 5- nutrition; 6- friction and shear. Each subscale describes the characteristics of what is being evaluated and receives a score that varies from 1 to 4 points in the first five subscales and from 1 to 3 in the sixth. Adding up all the points gives a minimum score of 6 and a maximum of 23 points. Anyone who obtains a score less than or equal to 9 points indicates that they have a very high risk for developing the injury, from 10 to 12 high risk, from 13 to 14 moderate risk, from 15 to 18 at risk and patients who present a value greater than or equal to 19 points, are considered without risk for UPP (BRADEN; BERGSTROM, 1987).

Initially, studies carried out to validate the Braden Scale considered a score of 16 for the risk of PU in adults and the elderly (BERGSTROM et al., 1987). Later, the same authors carried out other studies with elderly patients, in naturally unstable clinical conditions or with impaired self-care and suggested a score of 18 as a cutoff point to classify risk (BERGSTROM et al., 1998). In this study, a cut-off point was not determined as an inclusion criterion for the research, considering that these were critically ill patients, mostly elderly and restricted to bed.

When patients completed 24 hours of hospitalization in the unit and met the criteria defined in item 4.3, they were included in the research and submitted to the initial assessment, carried out by the researcher and a nursing academic from the Federal University of Paraíba (UFPB), through anamnesis and physical examination, meticulous inspection of skin conditions and estimation of the risk of PU by applying the Braden Scale, recording the information in the instruments described previously. Additional data related to clinical conditions and other risk factors relevant to the object of study were obtained through records in medical records and through information collected directly from the patient and/or family members.

To carry out the physical examination, the neurological, cardiovascular, respiratory, gastrointestinal, thermoregulatory, urinary and integumentary systems were considered.

The skin examination was carried out at the time of bed bath to reduce manipulations, always with the collaboration of the nursing team to reposition the patient from one side to the other, so that he could be assessed bilaterally regarding the integrity and characteristics of the skin, and the presence of pressure relief devices.

When UPP was detected in this first assessment, at least twenty-four hours after the patient had been admitted to the unit, the medical record was observed to check in the SAE form and also in the log book, whether the patient already had the injury at the time. admission or whether it could have already developed in the first twenty-four hours of ICU admission. The lesions were then assessed regarding their stage of evolution, dimensions and characteristics, recording the information in the relevant instrument (Appendix III).

The patient's weight and height were also recorded, taking into account the information provided by the patient or family member , given that we do not have a bed with a scale in the unit and the difficulty imposed by the clinical condition of most patients in standing on a conventional scale. To classify the calculation of the Body Mass Index (BMI), the indices proposed by the World Health Organization (WHO, 2000), described below, were considered:

Table 1 - Body Mass Index Classification according to the World Health Organization (2000).

BMI	CLASSIFICATION
< 18.5	Low weight
18.5-24.99	Normal
25-29.99	Overweight
≥ 30- 34.99	Obesity

Regarding the determination of the risk of PU presented by the patient, this was evaluated in each domain of the Braden Scale, adding up the points and obtaining the total risk.

Second Phase: monitoring patient progress

This phase of data collection occurred 72 hours after the initial assessment of each patient, with the procedure repeated in the same time interval until the final outcome of death, transfer or discharge from the unit. Thus, every 72 hours, clinical and skin conditions were assessed, the presence of other factors relevant to the development of lesions was investigated, and the Braden Scale was reapplied to determine whether there had been a change in the risk score for PU, as recommended by WOCN. (2010), when they mention that risk assessment must be carried out when the patient is admitted to the service and repeated at regular periods or when there is a significant change in the patient's general condition.

These assessments took place in the morning, during bed baths and interventions by the Hospital Skin Committee and all information collected was recorded in Appendix III.

At this point in the research, an instrument composed of five parts was used: 1 - Risk scores for UPP, which recorded the risk for each subscale of the Braden Scale; 2 - Laboratory tests that are related to the development of UPP; 3 - Other risk factors relevant to the formation of UPPs; 4 - Skin conditions; 5 - Assessment of the injury, which was intended for the clinical examination of pressure ulcers that developed after admission to the unit (Appendix IV).

To facilitate the recording of risk factors relevant to the formation of UPPs in the instrument, a list of codes was created by assigning a sequential number to each of the variables.

For laboratory tests, the values used by the laboratory of the institution where the data were collected were considered as a reference, which follows the values indicated by the reagents from the Wiener laboratory in Argentina. Normal blood glucose of 74 to 106 mg/dl; leukocytes from 3600 to 11000mm3; albumin from 3.5 to 4.8g/dl; lymphocytes from 20 to 45%, hemoglobin from 11.8 to 16.7 mg/dl and hematocrit from 35 to 49%.

Regarding the assessment of ulcers that developed after admission to the unit, the instrument items were extracted and adapted from the **"Wound Carrier Assessment Form",** developed by the leaders of the Wound Treatment Study and Research Group (GEPEFE) from the Federal University of Paraíba (UFPB), who authorized its use (Annex I). From the original instrument, items related to injury assessment were used, with those related to acute wounds being removed. In the chronic wound type, only the UPP item and its characteristics, dimensions and stages were selected, to which two more sizing categories were added, non-stageable UPP and suspected deep tissue injury, indicated by NPUAP (2009).

To evaluate the characteristics of the injuries, the international recommendations proposed by the NPUAP (2009) were recommended, which include grade, stage or category I, II, III, IV, non-stageable UPP and suspicion of deep tissue injury.

When a hyperemic area was identified, the patient was repositioned and after 30 minutes a new assessment of the area was carried out to diagnose or not UPP in stage I. In confirmed cases, the researcher herself called the Skin Committee for the necessary interventions. and also notified the nurse on duty to record in the service forms and other conduct pertinent to the team.

Ulcers in other stages were measured using a millimeter ruler, using the method of determining the greatest length and greatest width, regardless of the shape of the wound (IRION, 2012). It was not necessary to measure the depth of any lesion, given the non-development of stage III or IV PU. Data collection was terminated upon discharge, transfer, death or completion of the time determined for collection, considered as an outcome information from the last assessment carried out.

4.5 Ethical aspects

Before the study was operational, permission was requested from the institution's Administrative Director by signing the letter of Consent (Annex IV). The research project was then forwarded to the Research Ethics Committee (CEP) of the Federal University of Paraíba, complying with the guidelines of the National Research Ethics Commission (CONEP), contained in Resolution 196/96 of the National Health Council, which deals with research involving human beings, receiving a favorable opinion, according to opinion no. 023/12 (Annex I).

4.6 Data Analysis

The collected data were entered into Microsoft Excel and subsequently transferred to the statistical software PASW Statistic version 18 (formerly SPSS). After cleaning and criticizing the database, the results were generated through the application of two statistical techniques: Descriptive and Exploratory Analysis and Chi-square Association Tests and Fisher's exact in their simple and widespread.

The first technique is based on the construction of graphs and tables of simple or crossed frequencies when the variables of interest are qualitative, such as, for example, sex and marital status; and means, minimums, maximums and standard deviations are calculated when the variables of interest are quantitative. (BUSSAB; MORETTIN, 2006).

Based on the data collected, the incidence and prevalence of PU in the ICU was studied. From an epidemiological point of view, incidence refers to the proportion of people who develop a certain disease during the study investigation period, in relation to those who are at risk, while prevalence is the proportion of people who are sick in relation to the total that are at risk (ALMEIDA FILHO; ROUQUAYROL, 2006).

Thus, the incidence of UPP is determined by the number of new cases in a population at risk, in a given period of time, consisting of the number of patients who did not have UPP installed upon admission to the ICU and who developed them within the period of time for data collection, in the population exposed to the risk of acquiring UPP, calculated using the following formula:

Incidence index : $$\frac{\text{Number of new cases of a disease in a given location and time}}{\text{Number of people exposed to risk in the same place and period}} \times 100$$

Prevalence is defined as the relationship between the number of existing cases of a disease in a given population. In this study, Periodic Prevalence was raised, which measures the number of existing cases of a disease in a given period of time (ALMEIDA FILHO; ROUQUAYROL, 2006). The prevalence calculation was obtained using the following formula:

Prevalence index: $$\frac{\text{Number of new and old cases of a disease}}{\text{Number of patients in the population exposed to risk}} \times 100$$

Data to calculate incidence and prevalence were collected during three consecutive months of data collection (July 17 to October 17, 2012), extending for another 03 (three) days to meet the inclusion criteria that established that all patients underwent at least two assessments (initial assessment and one more).

The Chi-square Association Test and Fisher's exact test were used to examine the associations between the development of pressure ulcers (PUU) and sociodemographic and clinical data, as well as other risk factors for PU. According to Vieira and Hossne (1998), these tests are useful for investigating possible associations between two categorical variables.

To measure the association between two variables, a contingency table is used that describes the joint observed frequencies of these variables. Essentially, association tests compare the observed and expected frequencies, the latter being calculated under the hypothesis of independence (lack of association) between the variables (AZEN; WALKER, 2011). Among the association tests, the Chi-square test is the most famous. Despite being considered a non-parametric procedure, that is, a statistical technique that does not depend on the specification of any probability structure in relation to the data, the Chi- **square test has as one of its main "obstacles" the requirements regarding to the observed and expected frequencies** of the cells that make up the contingency table, such as:

- The table must not contain zero observed frequencies;
- More than 80% of all frequencies observed in the table must be greater than 5;
- The expected frequencies for the table must be greater than 5;

For large studies, in which the samples examined are greater than 200, 300 or 500 records, the chance of violating any of the above conditions is very small. However, for simpler and more realistic scientific experiments, in which the samples are small, one often encounters situations in which the Chi-square tests showed significant results, but, unfortunately, the researcher did not

may use them because one or more conditions of validity and applicability of the test were not met.

For these situations, it is necessary to seek alternative procedures that do not require so many applicability conditions. One of these procedures is Fisher's Exact Test (FISHER, 1934). Fisher's significance test is used to analyze contingency tables. Although it has been used in practice to study small samples (n *2* 20), it is valid for all sample sizes. **The test is said to be "exact" because the** probability calculations, coming from the contingency tables, are carried out based on their exact distributions and, therefore, do not depend on approximations for probability distributions when the sample size grows to infinity, that is, when it is very large.

Despite its great usefulness and practicality, a limitation of Fisher's exact test was its application only in 2*2 type contingency tables. Freeman and Halton (1951) proposed a generalization of Fisher's exact test, in order to expand its application to contingency tables of the R*C type (R rows and C columns). The principle of the Freeman-Halton test, or also called the Generalized Fisher Test, is the same as the Fisher exact test.

Therefore, in this analysis, Fisher's exact test will be applied, in its simple and generalized versions, to measure the associations between the variables, both replacing the chi-square association test for those situations in which its assumptions are violated.

It should be noted that the descriptive and inferential analyzes of the data were carried out through the assistance of a statistician.

CHAPTER 5

RESULTS

Considering the factors that may predispose ICU patients to developing PU, we sought to identify the incidence and prevalence of this condition, evaluating the risk score using the Braden Scale and relating it to the development of pressure ulcers, also checking the association between the sociodemographic and clinical profile and risk factors with the development of PU, with the results presented in tables and graphs.

5.1 INCIDENCE AND PREVALENCE OF PRESSURE ULCERS AND SOCIODEMOGRAPHIC DATA

To calculate the incidence, 36 patients were considered who were admitted to the ICU without UPP and who were evaluated at least twice (the initial evaluation and one more) and for prevalence, 45 patients who were at risk were considered.

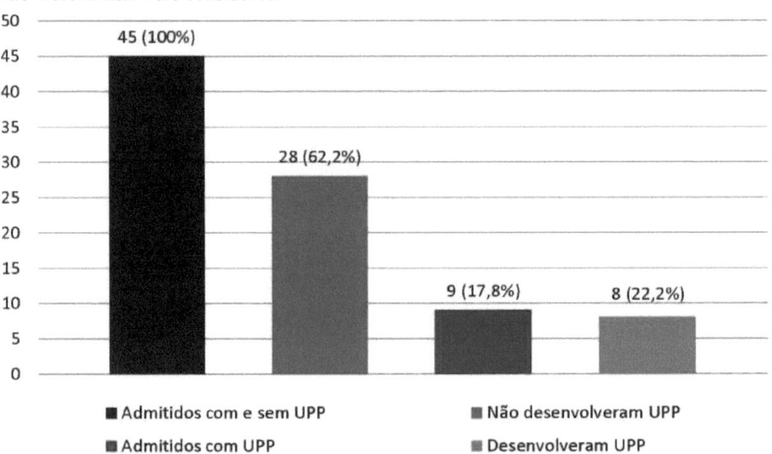

Graph 1 - Prevalence of pressure ulcers among study patients. João Pessoa - PB, 2013.

Source: direct research. João Pessoa — PB, 2013.

As seen in Graph 1, of the 45 patients participating in the study, 09 already had the injury and 08 developed it during their stay in the unit, totaling 17 patients with UPP, resulting in a prevalence of 37.8%. Among the 9 patients who were already admitted with the injury, there was no incidence of new ulcers.

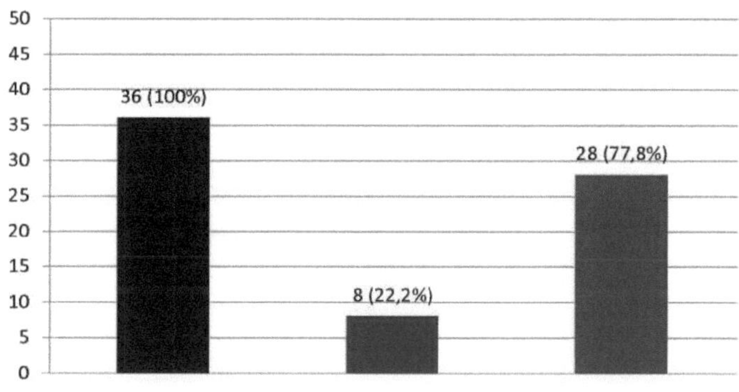

Graph 2 - Incidence of pressure ulcers among study patients. João Pessoa - PB, 2013.

Source: direct research. João Pessoa — PB, 2013.

As seen in Graph 2, of the 36 patients who were admitted to the unit without a UPP, 08 developed it during hospitalization, representing an incidence of 22.2%.

Table 1 - Sociodemographic profile of patients admitted with and without pressure ulcers. João Pessoa -PB, 2013. (N=45).

Variables	UPP				. Association Test (p-value)
	Yes (n=17)		No (n=28)		
	n	%	n	%	
Sex					
Feminine	6	35.3	11	64.7	
Masculine	1	39.3	17	60.7	p $^{(1)}$=0.7888
	1				
Color/Breed					
White	9	36.0	16	64.0	
Black	6	50.0	6	50.0	p $^{(3)}$=0.4949
	t				
Brown	wo	33.3	6	66.7	
Age group (in years)					
Up to 50	6	40.0	9	60.0	
Between 51 to 70	4	33.3	12	66.7	p $^{(3)}$=0.3770
Over 70	7	50.0	7	50.0	

Source: direct research. João Pessoa — PB, 2013.
(1) Chi-square test
(3) Generalized Fisher's exact test

Regarding the prevalence of UPP in the sample, it can be seen in Table 1 that the ulcer occurred more frequently in males 11 (39.3%), black individuals 6 (50.0%) and in the age group over 70 years 7 (50.0%). The Chi-square test and the generalized Fisher's exact test did not reveal a significant association between patients who developed or did not develop UPP, based on the sociodemographic variables analyzed.

Table 2 - Sociodemographic profile of patients according to the development of pressure ulcers after admission to the ICU. João Pessoa - PB, 2013 (N=36).

Variables	Development of UPP during hospitalization				Association Test
	Yes (n=8)		No (n=28)		(p-value)
	n	%	n	%	
Sex					
Feminine	4	26.7	11	73.3	p [(2)] =0.6940
Masculine	4	19.0	17	81.0	
Color/Breed					
White	5	23.8	16	76.2	
Black	3	33.3	6	66.7	p [(3)] =0.3961
Brown	0	0.00	6	100.0	
Age Range					
Up to 50	4	30.8	9	69.2	
51 to 70	t wo	14.3	12	87.4	p [(3)] =0.6193
7 70	t wo	22.2	7	77.8	

Source: direct research. João Pessoa — PB, 2013.
[(2)] Simple Fisher's exact test
[(3)] Generalized Fisher's exact test

In Table 2, the results presented show that there is no significant association, using Fisher's exact test, between sex, color or age group and the development of UPP. Regarding gender, a higher incidence was recorded among women 4 (26.7%), with the majority of new cases remaining among black people and people up to 50 years old.

5.2 - **Clinical data of patients with and without pressure ulcers**

In this item, in addition to the patients' place of origin, clinical data relevant to the object of study are presented, such as: underlying diseases, medical diagnosis at admission, medications used, physical examination, skin conditions, body mass index (BMI), laboratory test results, length of stay and time elapsed for the development of PU, considering the set of patients followed up in the unit (45) and the prevalence of PU for each variable studied. Regarding the time elapsed for the emergence of UPP, only new cases of the 8 patients in the incidence analysis were analyzed.

Table 3 - Distribution of study patients according to origin and occurrence of pressure ulcers. João Pessoa - PB, 2013 (N=45).

Place of Origin	UPP			
	Yes (n=17)		No (n=28)	
	n	%	n	%
Emergency/Urgency	11	45.8	13	54.2
Surgical ward	4	36.4	7	63.6
Wards	1	16.7	5	83.3
Other hospitals	1	25.0	3	75.0

Source: direct research. João Pessoa — PB, 2013.

Patients admitted to the intensive care unit are referred from other sectors of the hospital or other institutions through the regulation service. It can be seen that the vast majority of patients participating in the study come from the emergency/urgency service and the highest occurrences of PU are also observed in these patients (Table 3).

Table 4 - Distribution of study patients according to underlying diseases. João Pessoa - PB, 2013 (N=45).

Basic diseases	N	%
Hypertension	18	40.0
Diabetes Mellitus	12	26.7
Heart diseases	9	20.0
COPD	5	11.1
stroke	3	6.7
Others	18	43.9

Source: direct research. João Pessoa — PB, 2013.
COPD — Chronic Obstructive Pulmonary Disease; Stroke — Cerebral Vascular Accident; Others* — Leprosy, liver disease, myasthenia, chronic renal failure, neuropathy and Down syndrome.

Regarding the underlying diseases identified in the sample, the presence of one or more pathologies was found in 75% of the patients. As seen in Table 4, the highest rates were identified for systemic arterial hypertension 18 (40.0%), diabetes mellitus 12 (26.7%) and heart disease 9 (20.0%).

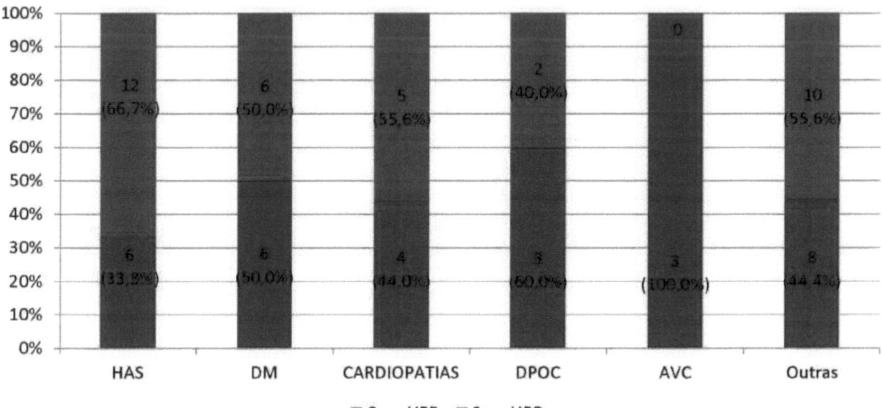

Graph 3 - Distribution of underlying diseases according to the occurrence of pressure ulcers. João Pessoa - PB, 2013. (N=45).

Source: direct research. João Pessoa — PB, 2013.

When analyzing the occurrence of UPP according to the underlying diseases, the following distribution is observed: 3 (100%) in patients with stroke, 3 (60.0%) with COPD, 6 (50.0%) with diabetes , 4 (44.4%) with heart disease and 6 (33.3%) with hypertension. There was no significant association by Fisher's Exact Test between the occurrence of UPP and the underlying diseases identified in the group (p=0.443).

Table 5 - Distribution of patients according to hospitalization medical diagnosis categories. João Pessoa - PB, 2013. (N=45).

Categories	N	%
Respiratory dysfunctions	26	57.8
Postoperative	15	33.3
Cardiovascular dysfunctions	11	24.4

Others	13	28.9

Source: direct research. João Pessoa — PB, 2013.
Some patients had more than one admission medical diagnosis
Others- Pancreatitis, digestive hemorrhage, pleural effusion, exogenous intoxication, acute lung edema and decompensated diabetes mellitus.

To facilitate the presentation of results, the medical diagnoses of patients admitted to the ICU were grouped into categories, with the most frequent being respiratory disorders 26 (57.8%) and cardiovascular disorders 11 (24.4%) and patients who were post-operatively (Table 5).

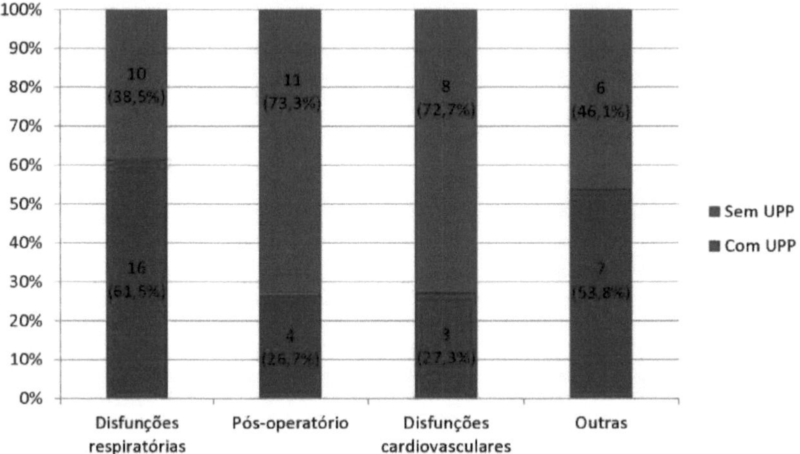

Graph 4 - Distribution of hospitalization medical diagnosis categories according to the occurrence of pressure ulcers. João Pessoa - PB, 2013. (N=45).
Source: direct research. João Pessoa — PB, 2013.

When analyzing the categories of medical diagnosis at admission and the occurrence of PU, it was observed that among patients who had some respiratory and cardiovascular dysfunction, 16 (61.5%) and 3 (27.3%) were affected by the injury, respectively. , and for those who were post-operatively 4 (26.7%). There was no significant association evidenced by Fisher's Exact Test between the categories of hospitalization medical diagnoses and the occurrence of PU (p=0.094).

Table 6 - Distribution of patients according to medications used. João Pessoa - PB, 2013. (N=45).

Medications	N	%
Antibiotics	30	66.7
Antihypertensives	15	33.3
Vasoactive	15	33.3
Corticosteroids	11	24.4
Others	5	33.3

Source: direct research. João Pessoa — PB, 2013.

The medications most used by patients in the study were antibiotics 30 (66.7%), followed by antihypertensives and vasoactive drugs which presented the same percentage (15; 33.3%).

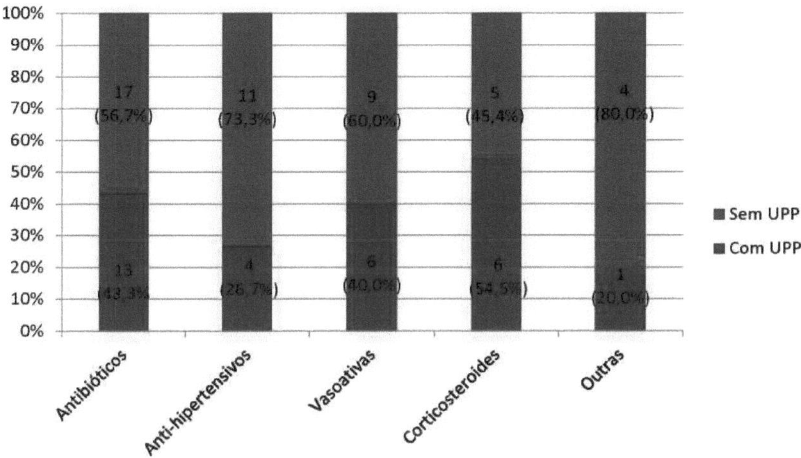

Graph 5 - Distribution of patients according to medications used and the occurrence of pressure ulcers. João Pessoa - PB, 2013 (N=45).

Source: direct research. João Pessoa — PB, 2013.

When analyzing patients with UPP and the use of medications, it was found that 6 (54.5%) used corticosteroids, 13 (43.3%) antibiotics and 6 (40.0%) vasoactive drugs. There was also no significant association between the use of medications and the occurrence of UPP through the application of the generalized Fisher's Exact Test (p= 0.574).

Table 7 - Distribution of physical examination data by system according to the occurrence of pressure ulcers. João Pessoa - PB, 2013 (N=45).

Physical exam	UPP				Association Test (p-Value)
	Yes (n=17)		No (n=28)		
	n	%	n	%	
Neurological System					
Lucid	1	5.3	18	94.7	
sedated	9	56.2	7	43.8	p [(3)]=0.000
Torpor/coma	7	70.0	3	30.0	
Thermoregulatory System					
Normal	15	34.9	28	65.1	p [(3)]=0.137
Hyperthermia	two	100.0	0	0.0	
Cardiovascular system (Peripheral perfusion)					
Normal	14	34.1	27	65.9	p [(3)]=0.144
Reduced	3	75.0	1	25.0	
Ventilation Mode					
Spontaneous	5	25.0	15	75.0	p [(3)]=0.135
Mechanics	12	48.0	13	52.0	

Source: direct research. João Pessoa — PB, 2013.

Sedated - using sedative medications such as: midazolam and dexmedetomidine (precedex) p [(3)] Generalized Fisher's Exact Test

As shown in Table 7, when the patients' neurological system was assessed, it was found that the majority of those who had UPP were in a state of torpor or coma 7 (70.0%). Concerning the thermoregulatory system, the presence of hyperthermia was identified in 2 (100%) patients who had UPP, the others were normothermic. Regarding peripheral perfusion, it was found that among patients with reduced perfusion, 3 (75.0%) had UPP. Regarding the ventilation modality used by the patients investigated, spontaneous ventilation prevailed for the group without UPP 15 (75.0%) and mechanical ventilation for those with UPP 12 (48.0%).

Table 8 - Skin conditions according to the occurrence of pressure ulcers. João Pessoa - PB, 2013 (N=45).

Skin Conditions	UPP				. Association Test (p-value)
	Yes (n=17)		No (n=28)		
	n	%	n	%	
Integumentary System: Hydration					
Normal	13	31.7	28	68.3	
Dry	two	100.0	0	0.0	P (3)=0.016
Peeled	two	100.0	0	0.0	
Integumentary System: Texture					
Thin or delicate	9	56.2	7	43.8	
Thick	3	75.0	1	25.0	
Lisa	5	20.8	19	79.2	P (3)=0.025
Rough	0	0.0	1	100.0	
Integumentary System: Tugor and Elasticity					
Normal	8	27.6	21	72.4	
Decreased	9	56.3	7	43.7	(3) P ()=0.107
Integumentary System: Edema					
Yes	4	36.4	7	63.6	
Anasarca	two	50.0	two	50.0	P (3)=0.896
No	11	36.7	19	63.3	

Source: direct research. João Pessoa — PB, 2013. p (3) Generalized Fisher's Exact Test

In the initial assessment, the skin of patients who did not have UPP was predominantly hydrated 28 (68.3%), smooth 19 (79.2%), with normal turgor and elasticity 21 (75.0%) and without edema 19 (63.3%). In those who presented changes in the skin's characteristics regarding hydration, all presented UPP (2;100% for dry skin and the same percentage for peeling skin). Analyzing the other characteristics of the skin of patients with UPP, it was found to be thick in 3 (75.0%), turgor and elasticity decreased in 9 (56.3%) and 2 (50.0%) in anasarca.

Table 9 - Distribution of patients according to Body Mass Index (BMI) and the occurrence of pressure ulcers. João Pessoa - PB, 2013 (N=45).

Categories	UPP			
	Yes (n=17)		No (n=28)	
	n	%	n	%
Low weight	0	0.0	tw o	100.0
Normal	9	37.5	15	62.5
Overweight	6	46.2	7	53.8

Obesity	2	33.3	4	66.7
Total	17	37.8	28	62.2

Source: direct research. João Pessoa — PB, 2013.

As shown in Table 9 , the calculation of the body mass index of the majority of patients without UPP revealed that they were within the parameters considered normal 15 (62.5%). Regarding patients with UPP, 6 (46.2%) were classified in the overweight category and 9 (37.5%) in the normal category.

Table 10 - Distribution of patients according to laboratory tests and the occurrence of pressure ulcers. João Pessoa - PB, 2013 (N=45).

Exams	UPP				Association Test. (p-value)
	Yes (n=17)		No (n=28)		
Laboratories	n	%	n	%	
Hemoglobin					
Normal	6	30.0	14	70.0	
< 11mg/dl	11	44.0	14	56.0	p [(1)]=0.335
Hematocrit					
Normal	1	11.1	8	88.9	
Changed	16	44.4	20	55.6	p [(2)]=0.122
Blood glucose					
Normal	6	42.9	8	57.1	
Changed	11	35.5	20	64.5	p [(2)]=0.743
Leukocytes					
Normal	8	34.8	15	65.2	
Changed	9	40.9	13	59.1	p [(2)]=0.763
Lymphocytes					
Normal	two	40.0	3	60.0	
Changed	15	37.5	25	62.5	p [(2)]=1.000
Total Proteins					
Normal	two	22.2	7	77.8	
Changed	15	41.7	21	58.3	p [(2)]=0.447
Albumin					
Normal	0	0.0	3	100.0	
Changed	17	40.5	25	59.5	p [(2)]=0.278

Source: direct research. João Pessoa — PB, 2013.
[(1)] Chi-square test
[(2)] Simple Fisher's exact test

Table 10 shows the blood components and their associations with the appearance of UPP. Most of the patients in the study had altered hemoglobin and hematocrit levels, among these, 11 (44.0%) and 16 (44.4) had the lesion, respectively. In the glycemia item, it predominated for the group with UPP normal values were 6 (42.9%), and for the group without UPP, altered values were 20 (64.5%). Regarding leukocytes, it was observed that in patients with UPP the values were altered in 9 (40.9%), while patients without the lesion presented values within normal limits in 15 (65.2%). For lymphocytes, a predominance of altered values was observed for both groups 15 (37.5%) and 25 (62.5%).

Regarding the evaluation of proteins, in patients with UPP, altered values were found in 15 (41.7%)

and when the type of protein was specified, albumin was below normal levels in all patients who had the lesion.

Table 11 - Distribution of patients' length of stay and the occurrence of pressure ulcers. João Pessoa - PB, 2013 (N=45).

Length of stay (in days)	UPP				Test Association (p-value)
	Yes (n=17)		No (n=28)		
	n	%	n	%	
<10	7	31.8	15	68.2	
11 to 20	3	27.3	8	72.7	
21 to 30	5	55.5	4	44.5	P [(3)] =0.387
> 30	2	66.7	1	33.3	

Source: direct research. João Pessoa — PB, 2013. p [(3)] Generalized Fisher's Exact Test

Regarding the length of stay, it can be seen in Table 11 that among the patients who remained hospitalized in the unit for a period of less than or equal to 10 days, the majority did not have UPP 15 (68.2%). In those where the injury was present, 5 (55.5%) spent 21 to 30 days and 2 (66.7%) spent more than 30 days in the ICU. The average length of stay was 18.5 days for patients with UPP and 13 days for those without the injury.

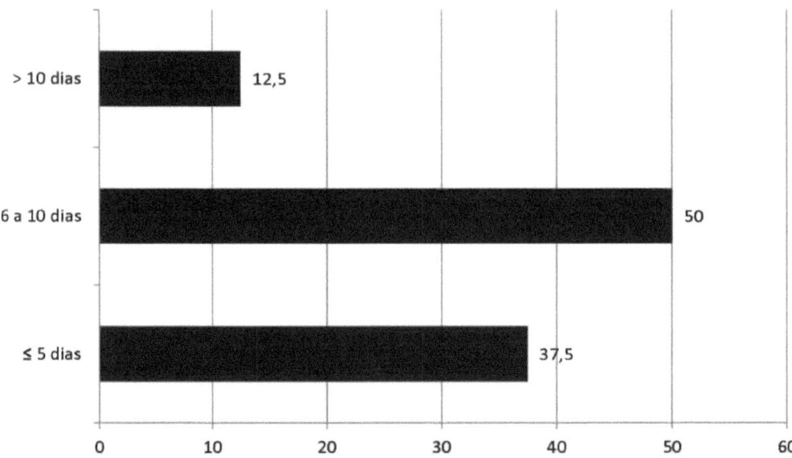

Graph 6 - Time elapsed for the development of pressure ulcers after admission to the hospital ICU. João Pessoa - PB, 2013 (n=8).

Source: direct research. João Pessoa — PB, 2013.

As shown in Graph 6, of the 8 patients who developed UPP after admission to the ICU, 4 (50.0%) of the cases occurred within a period of time between 6 and 10 days and 3 (37.5%) within 5 days.

5.3 Risk scores and the development of pressure ulcers

Patients were assessed for risk for UPP using the Braden Scale in the first assessment and in all reassessments that occurred every 72 hours during their follow-up, totaling between 2 and 16 assessments in the 45 patients.

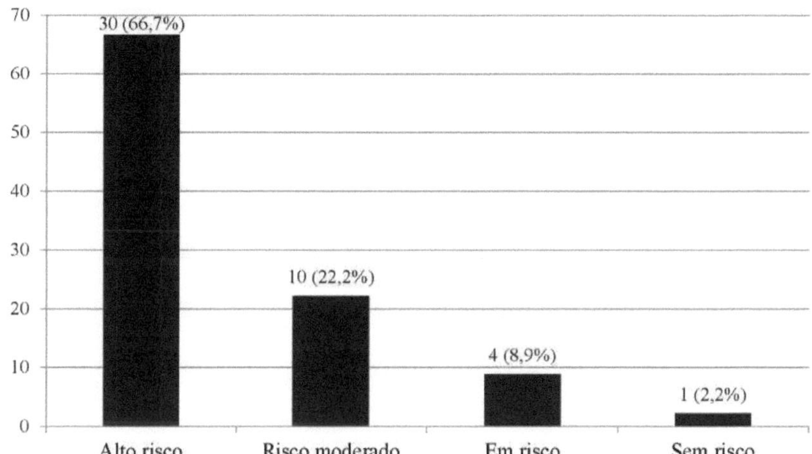

Graph 7 - Distribution of patients according to Braden Scale risk scores obtained in the initial assessment. João Pessoa - PB, 2013 (N=45).

Source: direct research. João Pessoa — PB, 2013.

It can be seen in Graph 7 that 30 (66.7%) of the patients investigated were at high risk (< 12 points) for developing UPP, 10 (22.2%) were at moderate risk (13 to 14 points) and 4 (8 .9%) at risk (15 to 18 points). Table 12 - Distribution of patients according to Braden Scale risk scores and the occurrence of pressure ulcers. João Pessoa - PB, 2013 (N=45).

Risk Score Assessment (Braden)	UPP				Association Test (p-value)
	Yes (n=17)		No (n=28)		
	n	%	n	%	
High risk	15	88.2	15	53.6	P (3)=0.093
Moderate risk	two	11.8	8	28.5	
At risk	0	0.0	4	14.3	
Without risk	0	0.0	1	3.6	
Total	17	100.0	28	100.0	

Source: direct research. João Pessoa — PB, 2013. p [3] Generalized Fisher's Exact Test

When analyzing the occurrence of UPP within each risk score, it was found that of the 17 patients who had the injury, 15 (88.2%) were classified as high risk and 2 (11.8%) as moderate risk (Table 10). Table 13 - Braden subscales and the occurrence of pressure ulcers. João Pessoa - PB, 2013 (N=45).

Domains of the Braden Scale	UPP				Association Test (p-value)
	Yes (n=17)		No (n=28)		
	n	%	n	%	
Sensory Perception					
Totally Limited	11	64.7	11	39.3	P (3)=0.114
Very Limited	3	17.6	two	7.1	
Slightly Limited	two	11.8	11	39.3	
No Limitations	1	5.9	4	14.3	
Moisture					
Very wet	1	5.9	two	7.1	

Occasionally Wet	16	94.1	24	85.8	P (3)=0.781
Rarely Wet	0	00.0	two	7.1	
Activity					
Bedridden	17	100.0	28	100.0	
Mobility					
Totally Immobile	13	76.5	12	42.9	
Quite Limited	4	23.5	9	32.1	P (3)=0.097
Slightly Limited	0	00.0	4	14.2	
No Limitations	0	00.0	3	10.7	
Nutrition					
Very poor	8	47.1	14	50.0	
Probably Inadequate	0	00.0	3	10.7	P (3)=0.481
Adequate	9	52.9	10	35.7	
Great	0	00.0	1	3.6	
Friction and Shear					
Problem	17	100.0	18	64.2	
Potential Problem	0	00.0	5	17.9	P (3)=0.016
No problem	0	00.0	5	17.9	

Source: direct research. João Pessoa — PB, 2013. p (3) Generalized Fisher's Exact Test

In the group of patients who did not have UPP on admission nor did it develop after admission to the unit, the most affected subscores in the **sensory perception domain** were totally limited and slightly limited, with 11 (39.3%) each. For the group with UPP, the totally limited subscore predominated with 11 (64.7%) and very limited with 3 (17.6%).

humidity domain , the majority of patients in both groups were classified in the occasionally wet subscore (16; 94.1% and 24; 85.8%). Regarding the **activity item** , 100% of the sample was bedridden, with the totally immobile subscore predominating in the **mobility domain** (13; 76.5% with UPP and 12; 42.9% without UPP).

nutrition domain , for the group with UPP, 9 (52.9%) were classified as having an adequate diet and 8 (47.0%) as very poor. For those without the injury, 14 (50.0%) and 10 (35.7%) were in the very poor and adequate subscore.

In relation to **friction and shear** , the most affected category for both groups was problem with 100.0% for those who had UPP and 18 (64.3%) in the group without the injury.

Table 14 - Distribution of study patients according to the use of devices and preventive care and the occurrence of pressure ulcers. João Pessoa - PB, 2013 (N=45).

Preventative devices/care	UPP				Association Test
	Yes (n=17)		No (n=28)		(p-value)
	n	%	n	%	
Support surfaces					
Pneumatic mattress	17	37.8	28	62.2	
Use of Devices/Coverages					
Transparent film	8	66.7	4	33.3	
Hydrocolloid with foam	3	50.0	3	50.0	p (3)=0.036
Transparent hydrocolloid	0	0.0	1	100.0	
No devices	6	23.1	20	76.9	
Position in bed					
Dorsal	17	41.5	24	58.5	

D, L [D	0	0.0	3	100.0	P=0.375
DLE	0	0.0	1	100.0	

Source: direct research. João Pessoa — PB, 2013. p [(3)] Generalized Fisher's Exact Test

Concerning the use of measures and materials to prevent UPP, it can be seen in Table 14 that 100% of the sample used a pneumatic mattress-type support surface (dynamic air). The majority of patients who did not develop UPP did not use devices applied directly to the skin 20 (76.9%), while among those who had the lesion, the majority used transparent film 8 (66.7%), showing a significant association between the use of devices and the occurrence of UPP. Regarding the position in bed verified in the first evaluation and considering the positioning in which the patient was placed after bathing in bed, the dorsal position predominated for both groups 17 (41.5%) and 24 (58.5%) with and without UPP, respectively.

CHAPTER 6

DISCUSSION

The harmful effects of pressure ulcers are undeniable and have drawn the attention of health professionals and researchers to the problem, which presents multifactorial causality and its occurrence is linked to the presence of some risk factors, affecting certain groups of more vulnerable patients, increasing morbidity and mortality.

These injuries are one of the most frequent complications in the intensive care unit as a result of the execution of invasive procedures and the greater need for manipulation, in addition to being critically ill patients, with associated comorbidities, restricted to bed and with limited mobility. movements and, therefore, more susceptible to injury formation (FERNENDES; TORRES, 2008; CRESMACO et al., 2009).

Everyone knows that UPP require multidisciplinary involvement to act from prevention to specific treatment, but it is the nursing team that has been demanding more action on this problem, which is justified by the profession's own work objective, which is consists of offering continuous care for 24 hours a day, especially in critical environments such as the intensive care unit.

In this sense, nursing needs to seek knowledge and skills to act with the various demands surrounding UPP, such as: knowing the causal factors and predictive scales validated and adopted by their institution, to estimate the risk that the patient presents to develop the lesion; master everything from wound physiology to techniques for measuring size and determining degree of evolution; and also recognize and know how to have the variety of materials available for the prevention and treatment of PU, in order to prevent the occurrence of this problem in their work environment.

It is of fundamental importance to carry out a diagnostic survey of the reality of the service through the incidence and prevalence rates of UPP, considering that they are important indicators to assess the proportion of patients who are affected by a disease or condition and develop it, at a given time.

In this investigation, of the 45 patients who made up the sample, 9 were admitted with previous PU and 36 without PU, with 8 of these later developing 11 injuries, representing an incidence of 22.2% and prevalence of 37.8%.

The incidence of PU found in the intensive care unit during the three months of follow-up of patients in the study, although still high, represents lower values than those found in some studies carried out in ICUs in public and private hospitals in Brazil. Matos, Duarte and Minetto (2010), when carrying out a study in the general ICU of a Public Hospital-DF, found a rate of 37.0% when monitoring patients for 2 months. In a non-governmental hospital in Santos-SP, 30 patients admitted to the ICU were monitored for 1 month and 11 (36.7%) of these had UPP (MATTIA et al., 2010). Another study carried out in an intensive care center of a large university hospital, in the interior of the State of São Paulo, followed 48 patients for 4 months and found that 62.5% of the sample developed UPP (FERNANDES; CALIRI, 2008).

Regarding the prevalence of UPP found in the unit, it is observed that the numbers are at the same level as the national and international scenario (37.8%). For example, a study carried out in the general ICU of a hospital in Portugal found a prevalence of 37.4% (LOURO; FERREIRA; PÓVOA, 2007). A similar finding was observed at the Hans Dieter Schmidt Hospital in the city of Joinville-SC, which analyzed 690 patients and found a prevalence of 41.5% for intensive care humidity (MORO et al., 2007).

These data reinforce that pressure ulcers continue to represent a serious problem within intensive care units, even with all the material resources and human training that have been sought to be imported into the units, in an attempt to reduce these numbers.

Analyzing all patients participating in the study in relation to the occurrence of UPP, it was found that there was a predominance of men, black people and over 70 years of age. These findings are similar to many studies in the gender and age category, but in race, the result differs from most of them. A prospective pilot study , carried out in an ICU of a University Hospital in Southern Brazil, found a predominance of males and white race in the group that developed UPP (BAVARESCO; MEDEIROS; LUCENA, 2011). Another survey carried out in two ICUs of a private hospital in Rio Grande do Norte also recorded the same predominance (FERNANDES, 2005).

Gomes et al., (2010) carried out a sectional study that covered 22 ICUs in 15 public and private hospitals in Belo Horizonte/MG, composing a sample of 142 patients and found 53.0% were male and 65.0% were male. those with white skin, but there was no statistically significant difference between these variables.

A study carried out by Anthony et al., (2002) with patients from various ethnic groups in the United Kingdom and mainly Pakistanis (non-white skin) and patients with white skin, did not show ethnicity as a risk factor for PU.

Regarding the age of the patients, even in the analysis of the prevalence of PU, the findings also corroborate those of Rogenski and Santos (2005) who found the average age corresponding to 70.3 years in the group with PU.

Regarding the incidence analysis, among the patients who developed UPP, there was a predominance of women, belonging to the black race and aged up to 50 years. Regarding the age identified in this group, the result corroborates a study carried out by Bavaresco, Medeiros and Lucena (2011), in an ICU of a university hospital in the South of Brazil, which showed an average age of 48.8 years for patients who developed UPP .

In our study, these findings are probably explained by the fact that patients who developed PU remain hospitalized for longer, using vasoactive drugs and corticosteroids and still have underlying diseases that are important for the genesis of PU, such as COPD and diabetes.

However, it is important to reinforce that the literature refers to the age factor as one of the most important factors in contributing to the formation of PU, considering the changes that occur in the characteristics of the skin and subcutaneous tissue (ROGENSKI; SANTOS, 2005; FERNANDES; TORRES,

2008) .

No significant statistical difference was observed using the Chi-square test and Fisher's exact test ($p<0.05$) between the sociodemographic variables and the occurrence of PU.

Regarding the origin of the patients who presented UPP, the majority of them came from the institution's own emergency/emergency department. Drawing attention to possible failures in the application of preventive measures in this sector, where patients who are recommended to be removed to the ICU often wait a few days until a bed appears to receive them, and it is up to management to reflect on alternatives that can minimize these problems. .

It has been reported by the media that the lack of ICU beds is not restricted to the institution under study, but is a reality in the daily lives of Brazilian hospitals, posing challenges for professionals who provide care to these seriously ill patients, in inadequate environments, and for the authorities, who have the duty to provide policies aimed at the comprehensive health of citizens.

Within the scope of the researched institution, one could think about increasing the number of beds, making agreements with other hospitals to receive critically ill patients, and if these are impossible, improving the structure of the red room (located in the emergency/urgency sector, where the the most seriously ill patients, sometimes requiring an ICU stay) providing support devices for the beds, such as the egg crate mattress, hydrocolloids with foam in areas of bony prominences and, mainly, raising the team's awareness of the complexity of the problem.

It is also emphasized that the nature of care in an emergency room is completely different from that in an ICU. The primary objective is to save lives, with other measures, such as preventing UPP, taking a backseat. However, with patients remaining in the sector, due to lack of space in the appropriate location, it is necessary for other interventions to be implemented to provide comprehensive care, which the Unified Health System (SUS) recommends in one of its fundamental principles (BRASIL, 1990).

In this scope, we see it as a great challenge for management to awaken in the team that works in emergencies the commitment and responsibility for implementing effective preventive measures to prevent this problem, considering that they are focused on another focus and that the structure does not cooperate to good accommodation and not with favorable conditions for the application of preventive techniques.

Concerning the underlying diseases, systemic arterial hypertension, diabetes mellitus and heart disease were the most prevalent in the sample. However, when investigated in relation to the presence of UPP, 3 of the patients with COPD (60.0%) had the lesion and among the 3 (100%) with stroke, all also had UPP. No significant association was found by Fisher's Exact Test (p-value < 0.05) between the underlying diseases and the occurrence of UPP.

These findings corroborate those found by Medeiros (2006) in an analysis of the prevalence and risk factors in hospitalized elderly people, given that the most prevalent pathologies were stroke 180 (60%) and hypertension 223 (74.3%).

Regarding the medical diagnosis at admission, respiratory and cardiovascular dysfunctions were evident in the majority of study participants with UPP. A study carried out in the Surgical Clinic, Medical Clinic, Intensive Care Unit and Semi-Intensive Care Unit units at HU-USP, found a predominance for the cardiocirculatory system (7 1.2%) and respiratory system (66.6%) (ROGENSKI; SANTOS, 2005) . In another study on factors associated with pressure ulcers in ICU patients, 54.5% were found for the respiratory system and 16.6% for the circulatory system (GOMES et al., 2010).

The cardiocirculatory system is responsible for regulating blood flow to the cells and when changes occur in the amount of this flow to less than the body's needs, there is a decrease in the supply of oxygen and nutrients to the tissues, causing ischemia, pallor of extremities and failure. in maintaining skin integrity (SMELTZER; BARE, 2005).

Therefore, these pathologies influence the formation of skin lesions in addition to interfering with several clinical conditions that can favor the development of PU (MEDEIROS, 2006). Fernandes (2000) highlights that these comorbidities are common in critically ill patients, causing hemodynamic instability and limitation of movement, requiring bed rest.

Rogenski (2002) adds that the impairment of the cardiovascular/respiratory system due to comorbidities and associated diseases, and continuous use medications, such as hypotensives, analgesics and corticosteroids, are also identified as conditions that influence the genesis of PU.

The medications most used by patients in the study are antibiotics and hypotensive medications. For the group with UPP, the most prevalent were corticosteroids 6 (54.5%), antibiotics 13 (43.3%) and vasoactive drugs 6 (40.0%).

A pilot study carried out with 74 patients admitted to an ICU of a university hospital, with a view to implementing the Braden Scale, also found antibiotic therapy to be the most used medication during hospitalization (48.6%), including among those with UPP (63.1%) (BAVARESCO; MEDEIROS; LUCENA, 2011). Medeiros (2006) also found that patients treated with antibiotics were the most affected by pressure ulcers 37 (12.3%).

The use of antibiotics can cause reactions such as maculopapular and erythematous rash, urticaria and edema at the injection site, fever, dyspnea and other systemic reactions that affect the transport of oxygen and nutrients to cells, interfering with the functioning of the body's immunity, leading to fragility. skin and vital organs (BONFIM, BONFIM, 2005). When it comes to intensive care units, the use of antibiotics by the majority of patients is explained by the increasing number of infections that have plagued ICUs in recent years.

Regarding the use of hypotensive drugs necessary to maintain blood pressure within normal parameters, these can alter blood flow and consequently reduce tissue perfusion and the tissue's ability to tolerate pressure (ROGENSKI, 2002). Fernandes (2000) adds that some medications, even essential for the therapy instituted for the patient, can cause changes in the body that lead to the appearance of UPP, such as hypotensive drugs, corticosteroids and sedatives.

In this context, Medeiros (2006) verified through a statistical test that there is a significant association between the use of medication and the occurrence of PU in the hospitalization of the elderly, an association not evidenced in our data.

When evaluating the neurological system between patients with and without UPP, a significant association was found using the generalized Fisher's Exact Test (p=0.000). Of the patients who were in a state of torpor/coma or under sedation (7; 70.0% and 9; 56.2%), the vast majority had UPP, while of the patients who had their lucidity preserved, only 1(5 .3%) presented UPP.

ICU patients are often under the influence of sedative drugs, which results in a deficit in sensory perception and difficulty in mobilization, consequently increasing the risk of PU (FERNANDES, 2005).

It is known that medications that act on the central nervous system, causing sedation, are widely used in critically ill patients for therapy or carrying out painful invasive procedures, but the effects of these drugs interfere with the patient's perception and mobility, making them stay for long periods. in the same position, increasing the risk of UPP occurring (FERNANDES, 2005).

Therefore, our findings are consistent with the literature when it mentions that changes in the state of consciousness are related to sensory perception, mobility and activity, which alone or in combination can trigger the formation of PU (BRADEN, 1997) .

In this context, the importance of early weaning from sedation and the use of all available resources to prevent these injuries is reinforced, considering the risk that these critical patients are exposed to, for the formation of this condition.

Regarding mechanical ventilation identified in the majority of patients with UPP 12 (48.0%), Costa (2003) mentions that ICU patients are generally connected to devices that make it difficult to change position. Fernandes (2006) adds that the use of these devices, in addition to pointing to a deficiency in tissue oxygenation, also causes greater difficulty in moving the patient and, consequently, a greater risk for PU. In the same research, the author mentions that she found a significant relationship between the use of controlled ventilation and the presence of UPP, diverging from our results, which did not show a significant association.

Regarding the characteristics of the integumentary system, recorded in the initial assessment, hydrated skin, with a smooth texture, with normal turgor and elasticity and free of edema, predominated for the group without UPP. In the group with UPP, the majority had thin or delicate skin, decreased turgor and elasticity, and anasarca.

Due to the longer hospitalization time experienced by patients with UPP, it was already expected that turgor and elasticity would be reduced and that edema would be present, according to other studies such as that by Fernandes (2005) who identified for patients with UPP, turgor and elasticity decreased in 70.0%, dry skin in 85.0%, rough skin in 70.0% and mild edema in 60.0%. Edema is a sign that can hinder circulation and interfere with the supply of nutrients to the cell, causing ischemia. It can be classified as discrete/moderate (+/4+), intense (+++/4+) and anasarca or generalized (SMELTZER; BARE, 2005).

Concerning the assessment of body mass index, values were found to be within normal limits for the group without UPP 15 (62.5%) and a higher percentage 6 (46.2%) for patients with UPP classified in the overweight category. However, these findings may not exactly express the reality regarding the BMI of these patients, considering that the unit studied did not offer a safe method for measuring the patients' anthropometric data.

A study that also addressed these categories carried out by Rogenski and Santos (2005), identified 42.2% and 46.6% , respectively, for the groups without and with pressure ulcers, classified in the normal category of the BMI table. Similarly, Fernandes (2006) found the majority of patients classified within the values considered normal and a higher average (28.6) for those who developed the injury in the pre-intervention phase, however, there was no statistically significant difference between the groups with and without UPP by the Mann-Whitney test.

In the evaluation of blood components, no statistically significant relationship was found with the occurrence of UPP, although all rates were altered for patients who presented the injury. The non-association may be due to sample limitations.

A case study evaluated **the "Monitoring Protocol for Critical Patients at Risk of Developing Pressure Ulcers" in patients hospitalized for a short period of time,** aiming to verify its effectiveness in patients hospitalized for a long period of time, and found in the patient monitored an average of 9 .38 mg/dl of hemoglobin, reducing to 7.8 mg/dl between the 13th [and] and 14 [to] week of hospitalization, coinciding with the period in which the injury occurred, leading the authors to consider the relationship between the hemoglobin level and UPP (ITO et al., 2004). The same authors add that low hemoglobin levels interfere with tissue oxygenation, increasing the risk of developing the injury.

Fernandes (2005) identified some predisposing conditions for the appearance of ulcers, including: anemia (90.0%), hypotension (80.0%), leukocytosis (75.0%), also noting that patients with leukocytosis presented a statistically significant difference (p=0.028) of 5.0 times greater chance of developing UPP, in relation to those with normal leukocytes.

Low albumin levels are also considered a risk factor for the occurrence of UPP (FIFE et al., 2001). Hypoproteinemia, especially albumin, can intervene in the prevention and treatment of UPP, as it is responsible for controlling the entry and exit of fluids from cells and when it is reduced, tissue edema occurs, which is considered an important risk factor for hypoproteinemia. presence of injuries. (MEDEIROS, 2006).

The reduction in serum albumin levels causes changes in oncotic pressure and, consequently, edema, compromising the diffusion of oxygen and nutrients to the tissues, favoring hypoxia and cell death (WOCN, 2010).

Regarding length of stay, it ranged from 5 to 39 days for the group without UPP and from 5 to 48 days for the group with UPP. The time elapsed for the development of the lesion predominated in the category between 6 and 10 days 4 (50%) and 3 (37.5%) within 5 days.

Bavaresco, Medeiros and Lucena (2011) found that patients remained hospitalized for a median of 14 (4-30) days and ulcers began to appear in the period between the 2nd and 26th day of hospitalization.

In the research by Matos, Duarte and Minetto (2010), half of the ulcers were identified between the 2nd and 4th day of evaluation, which reflects the reality also evidenced by Fernandes (2005), with patients admitted to two ICUs of one private hospital in Natal/RN, which detected 16 (80.0%) with up to 7 days of hospitalization. For Costa (2003), the development of PU normally occurs in the first two weeks of hospitalization.

In the first weeks of admission to the ICU, patients generally appear more unstable, requiring procedures to stabilize the clinical condition, with risk assessment activities and interventions for skin integrity taking a backseat (CARLSON et al., 1999) .

In this sense, patients who manage to go through this phase of instability without developing PU, but continue in this complex environment, bedridden, with changes in the level of consciousness, with impaired mobility, connected to devices, using vasopressors and corticosteroids, need to be seen by the team multidisciplinary group as a group at high risk for PU, and early prophylactic measures should be instituted, aiming to avoid

just the stability of the clinical condition and discharge from the unit, but also returning him to the family without iatrogenic complications, such as the much feared pressure ulcers.

Contrary to our results, Fernandes (2005), analyzing the length of hospitalization, found a statistically significant difference with UPP, revealing that the longer the period of hospitalization, the greater the risk for developing this condition. Cardoso, Caliri and Hass (2004) confirm the association between UPP and the period of hospitalization, as a risk factor for the development of this type of injury.

When measuring the risk for UPP using the Braden Scale, the categories of high risk 30 (66.7%) ($\leq$ 12 points) and moderate risk 10 (22.2%) (13 to 14 points) predominated. Other research found results with lower numbers than ours, but with a predominance of those classified as high risk for developing PU, such as that of Matos, Duarte and Minetto (2010) 55.5% and Silva et al., (2010) 57.3 %.

Analyzing patients with UPP 17 (100%) and the risk measured by the Braden Scale, it was found that 15 (88.2%) were classified as high risk and 2 (11.8%) as moderate risk, showing that the risk score is compatible with the development of pressure ulcers in these patients.

High risk scores for UPP are expected for patients admitted to the ICU, given that research results highlight this reality, such as those by Rogenski (2005) and Cremasco et al., (2009). This high risk is justified by the severity, complexity and condition of dependence that patients admitted to intensive care units are subject to (MATOS; DUARTE; MINETTO, 2010).

Therefore, the findings confirm the vulnerability of ICU patients, as well as revealing the importance of using the Braden Scale to predict the risk they present for developing PU, since the majority of them were classified as high risk, and of these, 15 (88.2%) had the injury, suggesting that this scale can be a reliable instrument to assess risk, considering the scenario, the population and the professional training of those who apply the scale.

Fife et al., (2001) investigated the Braden Scale as an instrument to predict the risk of PU in 186 neurological patients. Excluding stage I ulcers, they found an incidence of 12.4%. Braden scale scores ranged from 8 to 23 points and **patients with UPP obtained a score ≤ 15. With the exception of body mass index, the scale** was considered better than any other instrument for predicting the development of injury in the study patients.

Rogenski (2002), after finding data similar to ours in his master's thesis, mentions that these results allow us to confirm that the Braden Scale should be used as a predictive instrument for the risk of PU, both in the initial assessment and in monitoring the evolution of high-risk patients or even those who have already developed the injury during the hospitalization period, enabling interventions relevant to each case.

Scales are efficient instruments that can help nurses measure risk, providing support for planning individualized care, in order to intervene with patients with better results. In this context, Matos, Duarte and Minetto (2010) mention that for quality practice, care actions must be scientifically supported by the best clinical evidence, optimizing available human resources and reducing costs for the institution.

When searching for the most affected risk scores in the subscales or domains of the Braden Scale, it was found that in the sensory perception domain of patients with UPP, 11 (64.7%) did not react to painful stimuli, resulting in a lowered level of consciousness. or use of sedatives or limited ability to feel pain in most parts of the body, being recorded as completely limited. For the group without UPP, there was a predominance of totally limited and slightly limited with 11 patients in each subscale.

These findings confirm the need for care aimed at preventing PU in this group, considering that the sensory deficit that affects them makes it difficult to change body position or even request help to do so, increasing exposure to pressure and consequently to risk of developing the injury.

In the humidity domain, it was found that the vast majority of patients in the group with and without UPP were occasionally wet. It is expected that patients with a similar condition to the research participants will present dampness due to the lowering of the level of consciousness, restriction in bed, use of medications, dependence on hygiene and the edema that generally develop after days of hospitalization, leading to drainage of liquids through the pores.

It is important to highlight that humidity can be occasional, rather than completely wet or very wet, due to the fact that most patients use an indwelling urinary catheter and that the nursing team has some strategies to prevent the patient from being exposed to moisture. humidity for long periods, such as: placing a device for urinary incontinence in men, to channel diuresis to an external collector in those who are not catheterized; wrapping the exuding limbs with sheets and changing them when necessary, preventing this humidity from wetting the bed sheets, and routinely, the day team changes the patients in the morning during the bath and in the afternoon they check the presence of humidity, carrying out hygiene and changing sheets when necessary. The night team changes at the beginning of the shift and again in the morning, before changing the shift.

In the evaluation of Fernandes (2006), humidity was also not frequent in the patients in the study. The author adds that these results are probably explained by the frequent use of indwelling urinary catheters that generally occurs in the ICU, the need to treat some pathologies and strict control of diuresis.

Other research also carried out in intensive care units found a significant statistical difference between groups exposed to humidity or not, such as that by Fife et al., (2001) who found an incidence of 26.1% for patients with urinary incontinence. against 10.4% for those who did not have this problem (p=0.033) and that of Carlson et al., (1999) who also found a statistically significant difference between the groups.

Considering the seriousness of critical patients, which imposes many restrictions, as well as drawing attention to possible failures in material and human resources, in the activity item, 100% of patients were bedridden, meaning: not going to the bathroom, not sitting in a chair, nor in bed with legs over the side.

Currently, there is equipment (winch) that removes the patient from the bed and places them in the chair with the support and supervision of professionals. These data suggest that we need to evolve in this item, since we know the various risks that patients who are bedridden for long periods suffer, including muscular atrophy and the much feared UPP (FERNANDES; TORRES, 2008).

Concerning mobility, 13 (76.5%) of patients with UPP were completely immobile and 4 (23.5%) were very limited. Another study found the group with UPP (69.6%) to be completely immobile (GOMES et al., 2011).

According to the description of the Braden Scale, mobility is understood as the ability to change, maintain or support the position of the body, relieving pressure in areas of the skin/body, benefiting circulation. For intensive care patients, this mobility is generally compromised and is further aggravated by sensory deficits and comorbidities, requiring the team to plan geared towards preventing PUs.

An unexpected result was that of the nutrition subscale, which revealed that the majority of those with UPP 9 (52.9%) were categorized as adequate, that is, they received tube feeding or total parenteral nutrition (TPN). Strangely, in the group without the injury, 14 (50.0%) were categorized as having very poor nutrition.

The fact that patients with UPP are mostly receiving food is probably due to a longer length of stay in the unit, which results in stabilization of the condition and initiation of nutrition, given the benefits of keeping the patient nourished not only to prevent UPP, but considering the general context of intensive care. It is also emphasized that the genesis of these lesions is multifactorial, with diet representing just one more risk factor and not a determinant of their appearance. We therefore infer that these results are insufficient to relate or mischaracterize the occurrence of UPP with the food received by the study patients.

Analyzing friction and shear, the problem score was identified in 100.0% of the 17 with and in 18 (64.2%) of those without UPP, showing a significant association between these domains of the Braden Scale and the occurrence of UPP (p =0.016). Similarly, Fernandes (2005) verified the presence of the external factor friction and shear in 100% of patients with UPP.

These numbers are worrying and disturbing, because even though many authors share that this external factor contributes to the formation of PU, especially when associated with other risks, as is the case with critically ill patients, it is frequently present in our practice. The most aggravating thing is that the measures to eliminate this risk or mitigate it do not need many resources or new technologies to carry it out, they only require that professionals know the multicausality of UPP and commit to the patient and the service.

The movable sheet (known in practice as a crossbeam) must be used to move/transfer the patient, avoiding exposure to friction and shear, and must be adjusted to the appropriate position in relation to the patient's body, which helps to support the trunk, for elevation without dragging the patient when mobilizing in bed. In this sense, Wocn (2003) highlights the use of mobile sheets and skin-protective dressings as preventive measures that tend to reduce mechanical injuries resulting from friction.

In an analysis of the 6 Braden subscales and the related risk for UPP, it was observed that in patients who presented greater impairment in the categories: sensory perception (completely limited), humidity (constantly and very humid), activity (bed-ridden), mobility (completely immobilized), nutrition (adequate) and friction and shear (problem); a greater number of injuries were identified (GOMES et al., 2011).

The devices used and care provided to patients in the unit studied are similar to those found in other research carried out in intensive care settings in Brazil. A difference found was the use of a pneumatic mattress-type support surface (dynamic air) by all patients. On the other hand, although the unit has foam rollers, pillows and cushions to help reposition the patient in bed, frequent use of these devices was not observed during data collection. To reduce friction between bony prominences, such as between the knees and ankles, they use sheets, revealing that nursing professionals did not adapt the pillows made for this function, claiming that they are small and slippery, leaving the patient untidy, requiring the suitability of these devices in practice to be verified.

The devices used to prevent UPP in the unit are transparent film, foamed and transparent hydrocolloid plates, applied to the skin by the skin committee nurse. Checking the data collected in the initial assessment, the majority in the group with UPP used transparent film 8 (66.7%) and in the group without UPP 20 (76.9%) no type of protective device was used.

The transparent membrane or film is composed of polyurethane, impermeable to fluids and microorganisms and adhesive to dry skin. Indicated for the prevention of category I UPP, to fix and protect vascular catheters from contamination, protection of the skin surrounding wounds with exudate and as covers for intact incisions (SILVA et al., 2011).

The large-scale use of transparent semi-permeable film for the purpose of preventing UPP has been observed in practice, however, it is empirically known that this device does not contain components that function as a pressure reliever. The application of this film to areas of bony prominence may result in a lower cost when compared to hydrocolloid plates and foams.

Probably, the use of the film is important to isolate the skin and protect against friction and shear, but such benefits cannot be stated, considering that it was not the objective of our research, and other studies are needed to evaluate the effectiveness of these devices.

A clinical research carried out by Souza (2010) analyzing the effectiveness of transparent polyurethane film for preventing UPP in heels found a significantly lower incidence in the group that underwent the intervention.

It is emphasized that devices are important strategies in aiding prevention and as a fundamental complement to treatment, but they should not replace the implementation of measures that have been applied for a long time, and which do not depend on technology or high investments, but just a few simple and economically viable measures that can be used in both hospital and home environments, such as keeping the skin clean and hydrated, protecting it from humidity and friction and shear, changing the position at regular intervals according to the condition patient's clinic.

Regarding the patient's position in bed, the moment of the first assessment and the positioning that was carried out after bathing in bed were considered, verifying that 17 (100.0%) and 24 (87.7%) of the patients with and without UPP were in the supine position.

These findings reveal the lack of repositioning of patients in bed at regular intervals by the team providing direct care, neglecting the recommendations of the guidelines, which emphasize pressure as one of the most important risk factors for the development of pressure ulcers. Perhaps this attitude of professionals is related to the acquisition of pneumatic mattresses for all patient beds, mistakenly believing that since this support surface redistributes the weight, relieving areas overloaded by pressure, it would dispense with the ancient and exhaustive function of changing position. .

When researching these preventive measures and how they are applied in other realities, results similar to those of our practice are found, as seen in an educational intervention research carried out with nursing professionals from an intensive care center at the Hospital das clinics of the Faculty of Medicine of Ribeirão Preto/SP, which observed the position adopted by the patient at the beginning and end of the bed bath, verifying that the most adopted position was supine both in the pre-intervention phase 45 (90.0%) and in the post-intervention 44 (88.0%). At the end of the bath, 35 (70.0%) remained in the supine position in the pre-phase and 46 (92.0%) in the post-phase, that is, in the two phases and at the two different moments of the bed bath, the dorsal position prevailed (FERNANDES, 2006).

Fernandes (2005) found that among the extrinsic factors present in patients with UPP, the most frequent were: inappropriate type of mattress (density, time of use, thickness <13 cm) (100.0%), positioning in the same decubitus for more of 2 hours (100.0%) and shear/friction forces and pressure forces (100%), also confirming a significant association between these factors and the occurrence of UPP.

Once again, our practice is questioned, why have we invested so much in material and human resources to reduce pressure ulcers if we are not doing even the most basic things? Is there a lack of knowledge about the importance of this simple care? Lack of engagement? What can be done to awaken commitment and responsibility towards others in professionals? Is it work overload, since nursing is a profession with many activities during the shift? Are these questions restricted to the institution researched?

One thing is certain, the results presented here clearly express that we need to invest in educational actions that involve our professionals, making them knowledgeable about the problem, interested in solutions and sensitive to a more humanized and integrated service, which will certainly result, among other measures, in in the prevention of pressure ulcers and consequently in the reduction of incidence and prevalence rates.

CHAPTER 7

CONCLUSION

Considering the incidence and prevalence of UPP in the study, the results are similar to the reality described in some scenarios of intensive care units in Brazil, but portraying a lower incidence rate than that found in most studies in the same population. These data reinforce that pressure ulcers continue to represent a serious problem within intensive care units, even with all the material resources and human training that have been sought to be imported into the units, in an attempt to reduce these numbers.

A high risk for UPP was identified using the Braden Scale in most of the sample, with the predominance of the occurrence of the injury among patients categorized as high risk being consistent. The most affected Braden subscales for these patients were activity and friction and shear. In this context, the vulnerability of intensive care patients is noted, as well as the importance of using the Braden Scale to predict the risk they present for developing PU, suggesting that this scale can be a reliable instrument to assess the risk, considering the setting, the population and the professional training of those who apply the instrument.

The results allowed us to outline our reality regarding pressure ulcers and draw attention to the challenges we face in the face of such complex iatrogenesis, especially in intensive care, since even with all the investments already made in support surfaces, such as for example, the acquisition of dynamic air mattresses for all beds, the various devices for the prevention and treatment of UPP and the implementation of a skin committee within the institution, with a nurse and a nursing technician remaining within the ICU, there is still a long to do in our practice in order to reduce these numbers.

We recognize the great importance of new technologies from the perspective of preventing and treating pressure ulcers and we affirm that their benefits are undeniable in our practice, but we warn that we cannot be limited to these resources (even because they are often lacking in public services due to failure in planning and excessive bureaucracy) nor fail to carry out simple practices recognized in the literature as favorable to prevention, mainly because they do not require large investments and are contrary to the complacency of not carrying out care due to lack of material, since some of the most important for the prevention of PU, such as changing position, does not require any specific material to be carried out, but only the responsible involvement of nursing professionals who strive for the quality of care.

The results of this investigation will be shared with service professionals and the institution's management, so that everyone knows the dimension of the problem represented by pressure ulcers, strengthening practices that are being appropriate and reflecting those considered inappropriate, thus favoring changes in actions. of care provided in the researched unit.

In view of the findings and observations during the investigative process, the following strategy is suggested to reduce the incidence and prevalence of UPP in the unit: investing in professional training through ongoing in-service education and building and implementing protocols for the prevention and treatment of these injuries, a since there is some clinical research showing a reduction in incidence after these measures, which must be based on the best clinical evidence in order to help guide care actions, enabling better results.

REFERENCES

AGUIAR, ESS **Risk of pressure ulcers in elderly people with functional decline in physical mobility living in João Pessoa-PB.** 2011. 94 f. Dissertation (Master's in Nursing) – Federal University of Paraíba. João Pessoa, 2011.

AGENCY FOR HEALTH CARE POLICY AND RESEARCH, US Department of Health and Human Services. **Pressure ulcers in adults:** Prediction and prevention.1992, n.92- 0047.

ALMEIDA FILHO, N.; ROUQUAYROL, MZ **Introduction to epidemiology** . 4 ed. Rev. Enlarged. Rio de Janeiro: Guanabara Koogan, 2006.

ANSELMI, ML; PREDUZZI, M.; JÚNIOR, I. **F.** Incidence of pressure ulcers and nursing actions. **Minutes of nursing Paulista** . São Paulo, vol. 22, no. 33. p. 257-64, 2009.

ANTHONY, D, et al. Ethnicity in pressure ulcer risk assessment, with specific relation to the Pakistani ethnic minority in Burton, England. **J. Adv. Nurs** ., v. 38, n.6, p. 592-597, 2002.

AYELLO, EA Predicting pressure ulcer risk. Try This: Best Precautions in Nursing Care for Older Adults. **New York** , no. 5, revised 2007.

ARAÚJO, RD et al. Nursing and the use of the Braden scale in pressure ulcers. **Rev. infirm. UERJ** . Rio de Janeiro, vol. 18, no. 3, p. 359-64, 2010. Available at: http://www.facenf.uerj.br/v18n3/v18n3a04.pdf . Accessed on July 12, 2012.

FRIENDS OF THE GREAT AGE ASSOCIATION. Support surfaces in the prevention of pressure ulcers. **Aging and innovation magazine** . v. 1, no. 4, 2012. Available at: Http://www.associacaoamigosdagrandeidade.com/revista/volume-1-numero-4- 2012/superficies-de-apoio/ . Accessed on: October 14, 2012.

AZEN, R.; WALKER, CM **Categorical data analysis for the behavioral and social sciences** . New York, Taylor & Francis, 2011.

BAVARESCO, T.; MEDEIROS, RH; LUCENA, AF Implementation of the Braden scale in an intensive care unit of a university hospital. **Rev Gaúcha Enferm.** v . 32, no. 4, p.703-10. Porto Alegre, 2011. Available at: http://seer.ufrgs.br/RevistaGauchadeEnfermagem/article/view/17469/14445 . Accessed on: 12 September. 2012.

BERGSTROM, N. et al. The Braden Scale for predicting pressure sore risk. **Nurs.Res.New York,** v.36, n. 4, p. 205-210, Jul/Aug. 1987.

BERGSTROM, N. et al. Predicting pressure ulcer risk: a multisite study of the predictive validity of the Braden scale. **Nursing Research** , vol. 47, no. 5, p. 261-259, 1998.

BLANES, L. et al. Clinical and epidemiological evaluation of pressure ulcers in patients admitted to Hospital São Paulo. **Rev. Assoc. Med. Bras** . v. 50, no. 2, p.182-7, 2004.

BRADEN, B.; BERGSTRON, NA conceptual scheme for the study of the etiology of pressure sore. **Rehab**

Nurs, vol. 12, no. 1, p . 8-12, 1987.

BRADEN, BJ Assessment in pressure ulcer prevention. In: KRASNER, D.; KANE, D. **Chronic Wound Care** . Wayne, PA, 2nd edition , health management publications, p.29-36, 1997.

BRANDÃO, ES; SANTOS, JA; SANTOS, I. Compression ulcers: importance of client assessment. In: SILVA, et al. **Wounds** : fundamentals and updates in nursing. 3 ed. São Paulo: yendis, 2011.

BOMFIM, E.; BOMFIM, G. **Nursing medication guide.** São Paulo, Rio de Janeiro, Ribeirão Preto, Belo Horizonte: Atheneu, 2006, p.1-196.

BRAZIL. Ministry of health: National Health Council. **Guidelines and Regulatory Norms for Research Involving Human Beings** : Resolution 196/96. Brasília: Ministry of Health, 2002.

BRAZIL. Presidency of the Republic. Civil House. **Law No. 8,080 of September 19, 1990** . Provides conditions for the promotion, protection and recovery of health, the organization and operation of corresponding services and provides other measures. Available at: https://www.planalto.gov.br/ccivil 03/leis/l8080.htm

BUSSAB, W.; MORETTIN, P. **Basic Statistics** . 5th edition . São Paulo: Saraiva, 2006.

CAMPBELL, D.; STANLEY, J. **Experimental and Quasi-experimental Research Designs** . São Paulo: EDUSP, 1979.

CÂNDIDO, LC **Woundologist -** Interdisciplinary Center for Research and Wound Treatment. Available at: http://www.felderlogo.com.br/ Accessed on: 21 December 2011.

CARDOSO, MC de S.; CALIRI, MHL; HASS, VJ Prevalence of pressure ulcers in critically ill patients admitted to a university hospital **.Rev. Min Enferm. (REME)** , v. 8, no. 2, p. 316-320, Apr-Jun, 2004. Available at: http://www.enf.ufmg.br/site novo/modules/mastop publish/files/files 4c0cee7f70151.pdf accessed on October 15, 2012.

CARLSON, EV; KEMP, MG; SHOTT, S. Predicting the risk of pressure ulcers in critically ill patients. **American Journal of Critical Care** , vol. 8, n.4, p. 262-269.1999.

COSTA, IG Incidence of pressure ulcers in regional hospitals in Mato Grosso, Brazil. **Rev. Gaúcha Enferm.** v.31, n. 4, p.693-700.2010. Available in: http://www.scielo.br/scielo.php?pid=S1983-14472010000400012&script=sci arttext. Accessed on August 9, 2012.

COSTA, **I.G. Incidence of pressure ulcers and related risk factors in patients in an intensive care center.** Ribeirão Preto, 2003. 150p. D **issertation** (Master's) – Ribeirão Preto School of Nursing. University of São Paulo, 2003.

CREMASCO, MF; et al. Pressure ulcers: patient risk and severity and nursing workload . **Acta Paul Enferm, v.** 22, no. (Special - 70 Years), p. 897-902. 2009.
Available at: http://www.scielo.br/pdf/ape/v22nspe/11.pdf . Accessed on October 1, 2012.

CUERVO, FM Las Ulceras due to Prison: a preventable problem. In
Collection: **Nursing and Pressure Ulcers** : from reflection on the discipline to evidence in care, GRUPO ICE. Angra do Heroísmo, chap. 2 p.169-191, 2008
Available at: http://sociedadefeiras.pt/documentos/Enfermagem e ulceras por Pressao - Colectanea.pdf . Accessed on: June 7, 2012.

EUROPEAN PRESSURE ULCER ADVISORY PANEL; NATIONAL PRESSURE ULCER ADVISORY PANEL. **Prevention And treatment of pressure ulcers** : quick reference guide. Waschington DC: NATIONAL PRESSURE ULCER ADVISORY PANEL; 2009. Available at: http://www.npuap.org/resources/ . Accessed on: 10 Jul. 2011.

FALCI, JSP; CRUZ, ICF Risk assessment for pressure ulcer evidence based nursing practice. **Journal of Specialized Nursing Care** , North America, 01 Jul. 2008. Available at: http://www.uff.br/isncare/index.php/isncare/article/view/i.1983-4152.2008.1648 . Accessed on November 5th. 2012.

FERNANDES, LM **Pressure ulcers in critically ill hospitalized patients** : an integrative literature review **.** Ribeirão Preto, 2000. 168 p. Dissertation (Master's in Nursing) – Ribeirão Preto School of Nursing, University of São Paulo, 2000.

FERNANDES, LM **Effects of educational interventions on the knowledge and practices of nursing professionals and the incidence of pressure ulcers in an intensive care center.** 2006. 215f. Thesis (Doctorate) - Ribeirão Preto School of Nursing, University of São Paulo, Ribeirão Preto, 2006

FERNANDES, NCS **Pressure ulcers** : a study with intensive care unit patients. 2005. 139 f. Dissertation (Master's in Nursing) – Federal University of Rio Grande do Norte, Natal, 2005.

FERNANDES, LM; CALIRI, MHL Pressure ulcers in critically ill hospitalized patients: an integrative review of the literature. **Rev. Paul. Nurse** São Paulo, vol. 19, no. 2, p. 25-31, 2000.

FERNANDES, LM; CALIRI, MHLUuse of the Braden and Glasgow scales to identify the risk of pressure ulcers in patients admitted to an intensive care center. **Rev. Latin-Am. Nursing,** Ribeirão Preto, v.16, n. 6, 2008. Available at: http://www.scielo.br/pdf/rlae/v16n6/pt 06 . Accessed on: August 12, 2012.

FERNANDES, NCS; TORRES, GV Incidence and risk factors for pressure ulcers in intensive care unit patients. **Science. Care. Health,** vol. 7, no. 3, p. 304-310. 2008. Available at:

http://periodicos.uem.br/ojs/index.php/CiencCuidSaude/article/view/6484/3855 . Accessed on: 14 July 2012.

FERNANDES, NC S; TORRES, GV Ulcers of pressure in patients of intensive care unit: incidence and association of risk factors. **The FIEP bulletin** , Foz do Iguaçu, v. 76, no. 2, p. 55-58, 2006.

FERNANDES, LM; CALIRI, MHL; HAAS, VJEffect of educational interventions on nursing professionals' knowledge about pressure ulcer prevention. **Acta Paul Enferm, v.** 21, no. 2, p. 305-11,2008; Available at: http://www.scielo.br/pdf/ape/v21n2/a12v21n2.pdf . Accessed on September 15, 2012.

FERNANDES, NCS; TORRES, GV; VIEIRA, D. Risk factors and predisposing conditions for pressure ulcers in intensive care patients **. Rev. Eletr. Nurse** , v.10, n. 3,p.733-46.2008.Available at: http://www.fen.ufg.br/fen revisa/v10/n3/pdf/v10n3a19.pdf. Accessed on October 5, 2012.

FIFE, C. et al. Incidence of pressure ulcers in a neurological intensive care unit. **Crit Care Med Texas** (USA), v. 29, no. 2, p. 283-90, 2001.

GIOVANINI, T.; OLIVEIRA JÚNIOR, APG; PALERMO, TCS **Dressing manual.** São Paulo: Corpus, 2007.

GOMES, FSL; MAGALHÃES, MBB Pressure ulcer. In: BORGES, EL et al. **Wounds:** how to treat. 2nd Ed. Belo Horizonte: Coopmed, 2008. Ch.11, p. 189 223.

GOMES, FSL et al. Factors associated with pressure ulcers in patients at Adult Intensive Care Units. **RevEscEnferm USP** , São Paulo, v. 44, no. 4, p. 1065-71. 2010. Available at: http://www.scielo.br/pdf/reeusp/v44n4/en 31.pdf . Accessed on: October 10, 2012.

GOMES, FSL et al. . Risk assessment for pressure ulcers in critically ill patients . **RevEscEnferm USP** . v. 45, no. 2, p. 313-18, 2011. Available at: http://www.scielo.br/pdf/reeusp/v45n2/v45n2a01.pdf . Accessed on: November 11, 2012.

GOMES, AM Historical development of care practice in intensive care in Brazil. In: VIANA, RAPP; WHITAKER, IY and collaborators. **Intensive Care Nursing:** practices and experiences. Porto Alegre: Artmed, 2011. Chapter 01. p. 21-26.

GOMES, RC et al. Pressure ulcers: proposal for systematizing nursing care in an intensive care unit in the light of the literature. **Electronic Nursing Journal of the Center for Nursing and Nutrition Studies** [online serial], v. 1, no. 2, p. 1-18. 2009. Available at: http://www.ceen.com.br/conteudo/downloads/4552 31.pdf Accessed on: 08 Jul 2012.

IRION, G. **Wounds.** New approaches, clinical management and color atlas. 2 ed. Rio de Janeiro: Guanabara Koogan, 2012.

ITO, PE et al. Application of the monitoring protocol in patients at risk of developing pressure ulcers: a case study. **UNIPAR health sciences arch.,** v. 8, no. 1, p. 79-84, 2004.

JORGE, SA; DANTAS, SRPE **Multidisciplinary approach to wound treatment.** 3. Ed. Rio de Janeiro : Atheneu, 2005.

LINDOHLM, C. (20007), **Pressure ulcers with "case-study" in the Azores.** Available at: http://www.azoresglobal.com/canais/noticias/noticia.php?id=14056 . Accessed on November 22, 2011.

LISE, F.; SILVA, LC Pressure ulcer prevention: providing nursing tools and guiding family caregivers. **Acta Sci. Health Sci.** Maringá, v. 29, no. 2, p. 85-89, 2007.

LOURO, M.; FERREIRA, M.; PÓVOA P. Evaluation of a pressure ulcer prevention and treatment protocol. **RBTI,** vol. 19, no. 3, p . 337-341, July-September, 2007. Available at: http://www.scielo.br/pdf/rbti/v19n3/v19n3a12.pdf . Accessed on: 20 Nov. 2011.

MATTIA, AL et al. Pressure ulcers in the ICU: risk factors and prevention measures. **Public Health.** v. 7, no. 46. p . 296-299. 2010. Available at: http://redalyc.uaemex.mx/src/inicio/ArfPdfRed.jsp?iCve=84215678003 . Accessed on: September 21, 2012.

MATOS, LS; DUARTE, NLV; MINETTO, RC Incidence and prevalence of pressure ulcers in the ICU of a Public Hospital in the Federal District. **Rev. Eletr. Nurse** . v. 12, no. 4, p. 19-26, 2010. Available at: http://www.revistas.ufg.br/index.php/fen/article/viewFile/8481/8495 . Accessed on: 08 Nov. 2012.

MEDEIROS, ABF; LOPES, CHAF; JORGE, MSB Analysis of the prevention and treatment of pressure ulcers proposed by nurses . **Rev Esc. Enferm. USP** , vol. 44, no. 1 p. 223-8, São Paulo , 2009. Available at: http://www.scielo.br/pdf/reeusp/v43n1/29 . Accessed on: 20 Jan. 2012.

MEDEIROS, ABF Pressure ulcers in hospitalized elderly people: analysis of prevalence and risk factors. [Dissertation] [Internet]. Fortaleza: State University of Ceará; 2006. [accessed 10 September 2012]. Available at: http://www.uece.br/cmacclis/dmdocuments/adriana bessa fernandes medeiro.pdf

MESSER, MS Pressure ulcer risk in ancillary services patients. **Journal of Wound Ostomy and**

Continence Nursing . v. 37, no. 2, p. 153-8, 2010. Available at: http://journals.lww.com/jwocnonline/Citation/2010/03000/Pressure Ulcer Risk in Ancillary _Services_Patients.9.aspx . Accessed on: 21 July. 2012.

MORO, A. et al. Assessment of patients with pressure injuries admitted to a general hospital. **See Assoc. Med. Bras, v.** 53, no. 4, p. 300-4, 2007.

NOTES on nursing : a guide for today's caregivers. CABRAL, IE; GARCIA, TR (ORG.) Rio de Janeiro: elsevier, 2010.

PAIVA, LC **Pressure ulcers in patients admitted to a university hospital in Natal/RN:** predisposing conditions and risk factors. Christmas, 2008. 99f. Dissertation (Master's in Nursing). Federal University of Rio Grande do Norte. Christmas, 2008.

PARANHOS, WY; SANTOS, VLCG Risk assessment for pressure ulcers using the Braden scale, in Portuguese. **Rev.Esc. Nurse. USP** , São Paulo, v. 33, no. esp., p.191-206,1999.

ROCHA, JA; MIRANDA, MJ; ANDRADE, MJ Therapeutic approach to pressure ulcers - evidence-based interventions. **Acta Med Port** . v. 19, p. 29-38, 2006. Available at: http://actamedicaportuguesa.Com/pdf/2006-19/1/029-038.pdf . Accessed on: May 14, 2012.

RODRIGUES, MM; SOUZA, MS; SILVA, JL Systematization of nursing care in the prevention of tissue pressure injuries. **CogitareEnferm.** Niterói, vol. 13, no. 4. p. 566-75, 2008. Available at: http://ojs.c3sl.ufpr.br/oj s2/index.php/cogitare/article/view/13117/8875 . Accessed on: August 15, 2012.

ROCHA, ABL; BARROS, SMO Pressure ulcer risk assessment: measurement properties of the Portuguese version of the Waterlow scale. **Acta Paul Enferm** . v. 20, no. 2, p. 143-50, 2007. Available at: http://www.scielo.br/pdf/ape/v20n2/a06v20n2.pdf . Accessed on: October 14, 2012.

ROGENSKI, NMB **Study on the prevalence and incidence of pressure ulcers in a university hospital.** São Paulo, 2002. 109p. Dissertation (Master's in Nursing) – School of Nursing. University of São Paulo, 2002.

ROGENSKI, NMB; SANTOS, VLCG Study on the incidence of pressure ulcers in a university hospital. **Latin American Journal of Nursing,** v . 13, no. 4, p. 474-80, 2005.

SANTOS, CCV et al. Ethical and legal aspects in nursing care. In: SILVA, RCL; FIGUEIREDO, NMA; MEIRELES, IB **Wounds** : fundamentals and updates in nursing. 2nd ed. São Caetano do Sul: Yendis, 2007.

SERPA, LF **Predictive capacity of the Nutrition subscale of the Nutrition Scale Braden to assess the risk of developing PU.** São Paulo, 2006. 150 f. Thesis (Doctorate) - School of Nursing at the University of São Paulo, São Paulo, 2006.

SILVA, et al. Intensive Care Unit - ICU. In: FIGUEIREDO, NMA; SILVA, CRL; SILVA, RCL (Org.). **CTI** : nursing performance, intervention and care. São Caetano do Sul: Yendis, 2009. Chapter 01. p. 1- 42.

SILVA, RCL et al. **Wounds:** fundamentals and updates in nursing. 3rd ed. São Caetano do Sul: Yendis, 2011.

SILVA, EWNL et al. Applicability of the pressure ulcer prevention protocol in an intensive care unit. **Rev Bras Ter Intensiva** . v. 22, no. 2, P. 175-185. 2010; Available at: http://www.scielo.br/pdf/rbti/v22n2/a12v22n2.pdf .

SOUZA, DMST; SANTOS, VLCG Risk factors for the development of pressure ulcers in institutionalized elderly people. **Latin American Journal of Nursing** , v. 15, n.5, p. 958-964, 2007. Available at: http://www.scielo.br/pdf/rlae/v15n5/pt_v15n5a11.pdf . Accessed on May 15, 2012. http://www.scielo.br/scielo.php?script=sci arttext&pid=S0104-11692007000500012&lng=en&nrm=iso&tlng=pt . Accessed on: June 11, 2012.

SOUZA, TS **Evaluation of the effectiveness of transparent polyurethane film in preventing pressure ulcers in the calcaneus** . Curitiba, 2010. 95 f. Dissertation (Masters in Nursing) Federal University of Paraná, Curitiba, 2010. Available at: http://www.ppgenf.ufpr.br/Disserta%C3%A7%C3%A3oThaisdeSouza.pdf . Accessed on December 14, 2012.

SMELTZER, SC; BARE, BG Brunner and Suddarth: **Medical-Surgical Nursing Textbook.** 10. ed. Rio de Janeiro: Guanabara koogan, 2005.

OLIVEIRA, SHS et al. Development of pressure ulcers in patients admitted to a public hospital. In: IX BRAZILIAN CONGRESS OF STOMATHERAPY, 2011, Proto Alegre.

VIEIRA, S.; HOSSNE, WS **Medical Research** : Ethics and Methodology. São Paulo: Pioneira, 1998.

WADA, A.; NETO, NT; FERREIRA, MC Pressure ulcers. **Rev Med** v. 89, no. % p.170- 7. São Paulo, 2010. Available at: http://www.revistademedicina.org.br/ant/89-3/14- ulceras%20pressao.pdf . Accessed on September 12, 2012.

Wound, Ostomy, and Continence Nurses Society (WOCN). **Guideline for prevention and management of pressure ulcers** . Mount Laurel (NJ): Wound, Ostomy, and Continence Nurses Society (WOCN); 2010 Jun 1. 96 p. (WOCN clinical practice guideline; no. 2). Available at: http://www.guideline.gov/content.aspx?id=23868 . Accessed on 24 Jan. 2012.

Wound Ostomy and Continence Nurses Society (WOCN). **Guideline for prevention and management of pressure ulcers.WOCN** Clinical Practice Guidelines Series. Glenview (IL): WOCN; 2003.

World Health Organization. **Obesity** : preventing and managing the global epidemic - report of a WHO consultation on obesity. Geneva (Switzerland) WHO; 2000.

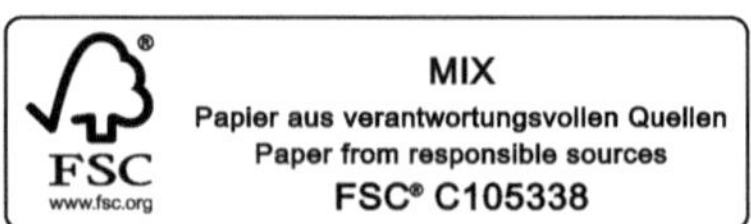

Printed by Books on Demand GmbH, Norderstedt / Germany